# Blood Results
## in Clinical Practice

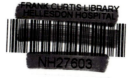

# Other books from M&K include

**The ECG Workbook 2/e**
ISBN: 9781905539772

**Preoperative Assessment & Perioperative Practice**
ISBN: 978190559024

**Ward Based Critical Care: A guide for health professionals**
ISBN: 9781905539031

**Practical Aspects of ECG Recording**
ISBN: 9781905539307

**Timely Discharge from Hospital**
ISBN: 9781905539550

**Mentorship in Healthcare**
ISBN: 9781905539703

# Blood Results
## in Clinical Practice

Graham Basten

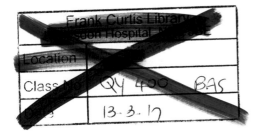
**Blood Results in Clinical Practice**
Dr Graham Basten

ISBN: 9781905539-73-4


First published 2013
Reprinted 2014

British Library Cataloguing in Publication Data

A catalogue record for this book is available from the British Library

Notice

Clinical practice and medical knowledge constantly evolve. Standard safety precautions must be followed, but, as knowledge is broadened by research, changes in practice, treatment and drug therapy may become necessary or appropriate. Readers must check the most current product information provided by the manufacturer of each drug to be administered and verify the dosages and correct administration, as well as contraindications. It is the responsibility of the practitioner, utilising the experience and knowledge of the patient, to determine dosages and the best treatment for each individual patient. Any brands mentioned in this book are as examples only and are not endorsed by the publisher. Neither the publisher nor the authors assume any liability for any injury and/or damage to persons or property arising from this publication.

To contact M&K Publishing write to:

M&K Update Ltd · The Old Bakery · St. John's Street

Keswick · Cumbria CA12 5AS

Tel: 01768 773030 · Fax: 01768 781099

publishing@mkupdate.co.uk

www.mkupdate.co.uk


Designed and typeset by Mary Blood

Printed in England by H&H Reeds, Penrith

# Contents

# Preface

This book is intended to serve three main purposes: **1**) as a supplementary text for under-graduate and postgraduate students studying nursing, healthcare, midwifery, physiotherapy, podiatry, biomedical science and medicine; **2**) as a working healthcare professionals' essential handbook for quick reference; and **3**) as a resource for patients and their relatives who may be keen to know more about what a particular test means. For ease of use, the text is divided into chapters that relate to the blood tests requested in practice.

*Blood Results in Clinical Practice* was written after feedback suggested that stories and analogies were very helpful to students wanting to remember the tests and their implications. Hence each section, where appropriate, contains an **analogy**, in addition to a basic overview of the relevant anatomy, physiology and biochemistry. It is therefore essentially an *aide-mémoire*, which links tests and conditions, and gives strategies for clinical practice using simple language and analogies.

Although the book contains individual chapters based on the usual blood tests, in practice these tests are rarely carried out in isolation. Instead, the results are like 'jigsaw pieces' that together build up a full picture, combining some results from the origin organ with some from other organs or conditions. For example, Chapter 3 discusses the full blood count. However, red cell number is partly controlled by the kidney so part of the 'jigsaw' for urea and electrolytes (Chapter 13) will be discussed in Chapter 3. In some cases, these connections are highlighted by the LINK ◀▶ symbol. Blood tests seldom provide a diagnosis on their own; they are best used in conjunction with case history, X-rays, scans and other reports by allied health professionals.

Given that reference ranges are specific to the local healthcare setting, and that the blood test should be interpreted against the associated range published by the healthcare organisation that performed the test, no formal ranges are presented in this book. The ranges used in practice reflect the local population, analytical machinery and quality assurance protocols in a particular hospital.

This book introduces common tests and common disease pathologies. It does not attempt to provide exhaustive coverage of all conditions associated with each test. Other pathologies may be present and should of course be investigated where necessary. Additional resources on other tests and related diseases can be found in the Further Reading section on page 76, and advice may be sought from your local pathology department.

The case study in Chapter 2 shows how the same tests can be used for many different purposes, and proposes a strategy for interpreting blood results. There are hundreds of possible underlying conditions so it was decided simply to present one 'all-purpose' sample case study, together with an interpretation strategy. There are other textbooks available that are entirely made up of case studies and these can be found in the Further Reading section. The case study is appropriate for training purposes only and is not transferable to individual clinical settings. Specific final diagnosis, prescribing pathways, treatments, additional tests and monitoring times are not included, as readers should seek definitive information on these aspects from their local clinical leads.

The values and interpretations offered in this book are based on current guidance from the National Health Service (NHS), the National Institute for Health and Clinical Excellence (NICE), the Institute of Biomedical Science (IBMS), the Health and Care Professions Council (HCPC), and personal feedback from colleagues and practitioners. Additional resources can be found in the Further Reading section.

For readers in the UK, local rules and regulations and trust procedures should take precedence over strategies proposed in this book.

Graham P Basten PhD MIBMS FHEA
*Head of Biomedical Science, De Montfort University, Leicester, UK*

# Abbreviations in the text

| | |
|---|---|
| **ACTH** | adrenocorticotropic hormone |
| **AFP** | alpha-fetoprotein |
| **AlkPhos** | alkaline phosphatase |
| **ALT** | alanine aminotransferase |
| **ANCA** | anti-neutrophil cytoplasmic antibodies |
| **aPTT** | activated partial thromboplastin time |
| **AS** | ankylosing spondylitis |
| **AST** | aspartate aminotransferase |
| **BNP** | B-type natriuretic peptide |
| **BPH** | benign prostatic hyperplasia |
| **CEA** | carcinoembryonic antigen |
| **CHD** | coronary heart disease |
| **CKmb** | creatine kinase mb |
| **COPD** | chronic obstructive pulmonary disease |
| **COX-2** | cyclo-oxygenase 2 |
| **CRP** | C-reactive protein |
| **CSWS** | cerebral salt-wasting syndrome |
| **CVD** | cardiovascular disease |
| **DVT** | deep vein thrombosis |
| **EDTA** | ethylene-diamine-tetra-acetic acid |
| **eGFR** | estimated glomerular filtration rate |
| **ESR** | erythrocyte sedimentation rate |
| **FBC** | full blood count |
| **FN** | false negative |
| **FP** | false positive |
| **GGT** | gamma-glutamyl transferase |
| **Hb** | haemoglobin |

| | |
|---|---|
| **HbAIC** | haemoglobin with glucose irreversibly bound |
| **Hct** | haematocrit |
| **HDL** | high-density lipoprotein |
| **HepBsAg** | Hepatitis B surface antigen |
| **HIV** | human immunodeficiency virus |
| **INR** | international normalised ratio |
| **K** | potassium |
| **LDH** | lactate dehydrogenase |
| **LDL** | low-density lipoprotein |
| **LFT** | liver function tests |
| **MCV** | mean cell volume |
| **MI** | myocardial infarction |
| **Na** | sodium |
| **PA** | psoriatic arthritis |
| **PE** | pulmonary embolism |
| **PMR** | polymyalgia rheumatica |
| **PSA** | prostate specific antigen |
| **PST** | plasma separator tube |
| **PT** | prothrombin |
| **PTG** | parathyroid gland |
| **PTH** | parathyroid hormone |
| **PV** | plasma viscosity |
| **RA** | rheumatoid arthritis |
| **RBC** | red blood cell count |
| **Rh** | Rhesus |
| **SIADH** | syndrome of inappropriate anti-diuretic hormone |
| **SLE** | systemic lupus erythematosus |
| **SPEP** | serum protein electrophoresis |
| **SST** | serum separator tube |

| | |
|---|---|
| **T3** | triiodothyronine |
| **T4** | thyroxine |
| **TIBC** | total iron binding capacity |
| **TN** | true negative |
| **TP** | true positive |
| **TRH** | thyrotropin-releasing hormone |
| **TSH** | thyroid-stimulating hormone |
| **U&Es** | urea and electrolytes |
| **ULN** | upper limit of normal |
| **VTE** | venous thromboembolism |
| **VWF** | von Willebrand's factor |
| **WBC** | white blood cell count |
| **WS** | Well's score |

# 1

# Understanding blood tests

This book will enable you to:

- Appreciate the importance of blood tests in diagnosis and patient management
- Augment your current knowledge by defining what each test is, and explaining what it shows from a physiological and biochemical viewpoint
- Understand the many abbreviations used in blood tests (see Table 1)
- Work through the case study presented in Chapter 2, and then seek additional relevant case studies from the Further Reading section and local sources
- Determine the clinical significance of values outside the reference range, or indeed of an ill person with normal results
- Develop linking of tests and using tests for exclusion
- Try out the strategy example in Chapter 2, adapting it to your own clinical setting
- Explore how tests form a natural hierarchy, with full blood count (FBC), urea and electrolytes (U&Es) and liver function tests (LFTs) being common first-line tests, which may then justify more specific (and often more expensive) tests.

## Quick reference glossary

The following table shows common terms, abbreviations and some typical observations relating to the various blood tests. Some examples also have metaphors, shown in quotation marks, to aid memory and understanding. These will be explained further in the corresponding chapters.

## Table 1.1: Glossary of terms used in blood tests

| Full blood count (FBC) | |
|---|---|
| Platelet | <ul><li>Cell that causes the blood to clot</li><li>Also a marker of bone marrow function</li><li>Decreased in some leukaemia and myelomas</li><li>Additional test is mean platelet volume (MPV)</li></ul> |

| | |
|---|---|
| White blood cell count (WBC) | • The total number of white cells in the blood |
| Neutrophil | • A type of white blood cell<br>• Responds to tissue damage via C-reactive protein (or CRP)<br>• Raised in bacterial infections, autoimmune conditions<br>• **'The fire engine'** |
| Lymphocyte | • A type of white blood cell<br>• Makes antibodies<br>• Raised in viral infections and some myelomas<br>• **'The police'** |
| Monocyte | • A type of white blood cell<br>• Infiltrates the tissue in systemic bacterial infections<br>• Linked to cardiovascular disease and high low-density lipoprotein (LDL) cholesterol<br>• **'The miner'** |
| Basophil | • A type of white blood cell<br>• Important in allergic responses and hypersensitivity |
| Eosinophil | • A type of white blood cell<br>• Important in allergic responses and hypersensitivity |
| Blast/Atypical | • A type of dysfunctional white cell<br>• Raised in leukaemia and myelomas |
| Haematocrit (Hct) | • Percentage of red blood cells in the whole blood<br>• Decreased in anaemia<br>• Elevated in polycythaemia |
| Haemoglobin (Hb) | • The oxygen-carrying protein in the red blood cell<br>• Decreased in anaemia<br>• Elevated in polycythaemia |
| Red blood cell count (RBC) | • The total number of red blood cells in the blood as a count<br>• Decreased in anaemia<br>• Elevated in polycythaemia |

| Mean cell volume (MCV) | • The average size of the red blood cells<br>• Low in iron deficient anaemia<br>• Normal in blood loss anaemia<br>• High in folate and $B_{12}$ deficient anaemia |
|---|---|
| **Inflammatory markers** | |
| Plasma viscosity (PV) | • A measure of more 'stuff' in the blood<br>• Thus, a surrogate, non-specific marker of<br>• inflammation<br>• Increased in autoimmune conditions, infection, cell damage, cancer, myelomas<br>• **'The traffic jam due to fire engines and police (white cells)'**<br>• Could remain raised for two weeks post-injury, as increased white cells have around two-week lifespan |
| Erythrocyte sedimentation rate (ESR) | • How quickly red blood cells fall in a tube, in a lab<br>• A surrogate, non-specific, marker of inflammation that has elicited a fibrinogen response<br>• Fibrinogen 'sticks' red blood cells together so they become heavier and fall more quickly<br>• Could be normal in low damage inflammation as seen in some autoimmune conditions<br>• **'The scaffolding and building-supporting structure following a large fire'**<br>• If raised, could remain raised for a significant time post-event |
| C-reactive protein (CRP) | • A chemo-attractant protein released in response to tissue damage<br>• **'The fire alarm'**<br>• Possible to miss the CRP response post-injury whilst still having raised PV and ESR<br>• Increasingly being used as a sensitive marker for atherosclerotic vascular damage to indicate cardiovascular risk |

| Urea and electrolytes (U&Es), Kidney function | |
| --- | --- |
| Sodium (Na) | • Extracellular electrolyte that controls water balance and blood pressure<br>• Raised in dehydration, ◀▶ urea |
| Potassium (K) | • Intracellular electrolyte, controls cellular pumps and receptors via electric potential<br>• Therefore a red flag if in high concentrations in the blood |
| Urea | • A marker of acute renal dysfunction, such as distress, although this could be something like dehydration, so ◀▶ to Na levels |
| Creatinine | • A marker of chronic renal function, such as a renal stone |
| Estimated glomerular filtration rate (eGFR) | • A general marker of kidney function<br>• Used to diagnose chronic kidney disease staging<br>• Used to confirm renal dysfunction as cause of other conditions such as renal anaemia |
| **Liver function tests (LFTs)** | |
| Alanine aminotransferase (ALT) | • A liver enzyme<br>• Often raised in trauma, drug toxicity, and viral hepatitis |
| Aspartate aminotransferase (AST) | • A liver enzyme<br>• Often raised in trauma, acute alcohol hepatitis and liver failure<br>• Also found in the heart so ◀▶ to cardiac markers/chest pain |
| Gamma-glutamyl transferase (GGT) | • A liver enzyme<br>• Often raised following alcohol intake<br>• ◀▶ to RBC, MCV and folate to differentiate between alcohol, $B_{12}$ and diabetes neuropathies |
| Alkaline phosphatase | • A liver enzyme<br>• Often increased in biliary tree damage such as gallstones<br>Also found in the bone (check Ca), kidney (check<br>• U&Es) and placenta (check age and gender) |

| Amylase | • A liver enzyme<br>• Often increased in pancreatitis and pancreatic tumours |
|---|---|
| Bilirubin | • A marker of the 'plumbing' of the liver<br>• Increased in jaundice, usually caused by pre-, actual or post-hepatic blockage |
| Urobilinogen | • A bilirubin breakdown product, usually absent in post-hepatic jaundice |
| Albumin | • A protein produced by the liver<br>• A chaperone for chemicals like Ca so could give false low value in nutrient-deficient patients<br>• Decreased in liver damage |
| Globulin | • A crude marker of antibody production/presence<br>• Often increased in autoimmune conditions, myelomas and viral infection |

**Additional tests**

| D-Dimer | • A breakdown product of a clot<br>• Care should be taken to link D-dimers to deep vein thrombosis (DVT) and pulmonary embolism (PE)<br>• Refer to NICE guidelines (UK) |
|---|---|
| International normalised ratio (INR) | • How long it takes for your blood to clot is given a baseline value of 1, thus an INR of 2 would mean your blood is taking twice as long to clot<br>• Goes up in anti-coagulation and liver disease |
| Bence Jones protein | • A breakdown product of a 'nonsense' antibody<br>• Usually present in a myeloma |
| Bone profile | • Usually returns corrected Ca, PTH and vitamin $D_3$<br>• Can help differentiate between osteomalacia (rickets), Paget's and osteoporosis |

| | |
|---|---|
| Prostate specific antigen (PSA) | • Released by the prostate<br>• Relative to prostate damage<br>• A slightly raised PSA may not mean prostate cancer<br>• Link to urea and Alk phos, and Ca (secondary bone metastasis) |
| CA-125 | • A marker of ovarian cancer |
| Thyroid function | • Thyroxine (T4), thyrotrophic releasing hormone (TRH) and thyroid stimulating hormone (TSH) are measured to diagnose cause of primary, secondary or tertiary hypothyroidism (or hyperthyroidism); additional confirmatory tests may be required<br>• Also used to titre T4 supplements |
| Autoimmune markers | • Rheumatoid factor (rheumatoid arthritis) and ankylosing spondylitis (HLAB27) are types of self-antibodies that are often present in autoimmune conditions<br>• Intrinsic factor and parietal cell antibody for pernicious anaemia |
| Haemoglobin with glucose irreversibly bound (HbA1c) | • A long-term marker of glucose in excess, used in diabetes monitoring |
| Acid Base pH Bicarbonate | • Used to monitor respiratory (chronic obstructive pulmonary disease) and metabolic (drug overdose) acidosis or alkalosis |
| Ferritin (Iron), Folate, $B_{12}$ | • Nutrient markers to be used with RBC, Hb and MCV<br>• Low MCV usually has low ferritin (high ferritin in hemochromatosis)<br>• High MCV usually has low folate and/or low $B_{12}$<br>• Low folate from sustained alcohol, drug interactions, diet or gastro-intestinal (GI) conditions<br>• Low $B_{12}$ from GI conditions, diet and autoimmune pernicious anaemia |

| Troponins, creatine kinase mb (CKmb), B-type natriuretic peptide (BNP) | • Cardiac event markers <br> • Troponins and CKmb are proteins found in the cardiac tissue that are present in high concentrations in the blood following a cardiac event <br> • BNP is a peptide found in the cardiac wall; increased levels may mean ventricular wall load is dysfunctional and may predispose to a cardiac event |
|---|---|

## Clinical implications of results and understanding reference ranges

Blood tests are placed in context by reference ranges. Patients often fall outside these ranges, yet there is little or no clinical intervention. In this section, we look at how some of these test results can be affected by blood collection methods. We also discuss the ways in which reference ranges are constructed and used.

### Blood collection and storage techniques

Tourniquets are often used to collect blood samples because they block venous return and cause dilatation, thus enabling easier identification of entry points. However, this typically causes loss of water and electrolytes from plasma, which may increase plasma protein levels. The stasis of blood flow can also produce different metabolic products (such as lactate); and if the patient is asked to clench their fist this may cause an artifactual hyperkalaemia (an elevated potassium level). These disadvantages do not mean that we should not use tourniquets. However, if results appear unreliable or unlikely – based on a patient's symptoms – it may be due to these factors.

Other problems include poor patient identification, samples taking more than 72 hours to be transported to the service, and samples being stored at the wrong temperature or not protected from light. To reduce the risk of these errors, each test has its own blood collection protocol.

### The difference between plasma and serum

Plasma is the liquid component of the blood. It is predominantly made up of water, but also contains electrolytes and some proteins, glucose, hormones, $CO_2$ and the cells that make up the whole blood sample. Serum is the cell-free liquid component of the blood after clotting has occurred; thus fibrinogen, cells and other clotting factors are not present. Serum is usually

sample. This will cause errors in reporting, for example, elevated potassium, magnesium and phosphate. The laboratory may be able to negate the effect of using a haemolysed sample if the result is needed urgently or it is difficult to obtain another sample. Common reasons for the sample being haemolysed include:

- the collection needle gauge being too narrow
- over-vigorous shaking of the sample
- an underlying haematological disorder
- red cells being isolated for storage and then stored in water or a non-isotonic solution
- over-vigorous dispensing of blood from the hypodermic syringe to collection tubes.

## Reference ranges

Most people are comfortable with the idea of reference ranges, but what do they actually tell us? Or, rather, what *don't* they tell us? To create a reference range, a number of volunteers (usually over 120) are matched for factors such as age, gender and ethnicity, and the analyte of interest is then measured. Firstly, most ranges have a 95% confidence, which means that the top 2.5% of values and the bottom 2.5% of values are omitted. In other words, it is possible to be healthy but outside the reference range because you are at the very top or the very bottom, neither of which are shown. Secondly, you should use ranges from unvalidated sources with great care, as ranges can vary with age and gender and local population. Best practice is to use the range that is presented with the actual value.

**Analogy: If you measured the height of 120 shoppers at a supermarket, the world's smallest man and the world's tallest man might be present and be included in your sample. However, it's unlikely that you'll see them again, so the top and bottom of the data is cropped, leaving more of the average making up the range. This is the first problem with reference ranges. Of the healthy cohort, around 5% are excluded at this initial stage, leaving them outside the range.**

### Clinical cut-off values

Reference ranges are generally used to identify a range of 'normality'. A value outside this range may therefore justify further investigation. Values outside reference ranges may be matched to case control studies. They can then be given a disease progression status, using clinical cut-off values.

**Example**: Prostate-specific antigen (PSA) is secreted from the prostate, and elevation may require further investigation. In a case control trial in men with benign prostatic hyperplasia

(BPH), normal and cancer (PC), PSA was measured and followed a trend:

0–4 ng/mL (PSA) = normal reference range

4–10 ng/mL = BPH but not PC, some normal

10–20 ng/mL = often PC

>20 ng/ML = almost always PC

## Clinical sensitivity and specificity

Because most blood tests have an associated pathology but may not be very accurate in detecting a specific disease, they sometimes produce 'false positives'. PSA is a good example of such a test. Clinical specificity refers to whether the test can correctly report someone without the disease as being 'healthy'. Conversely, clinical sensitivity refers to whether the test can correctly report someone with the disease as being 'diseased'.

The terms used to describe this are:

- True negative (TN): patient is healthy and blood test result is within reference range
- True positive (TP): patient has condition and blood test result is outside the reference range
- False negative (FN): patient has condition but the blood test result falls within the normal reference range
- False positive (FP): patient is healthy but the blood test result is outside the reference range.

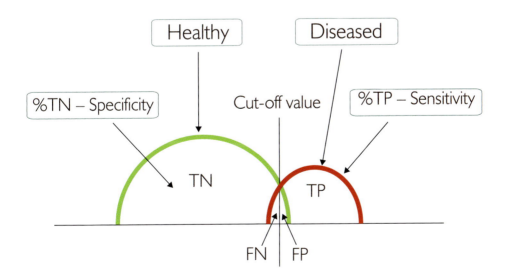

Figure 1.2: The cut-off value between 'healthy' and 'diseased'

The cut-off value is the point at which people change from being labelled 'healthy' to being labelled 'diseased', or the reverse. If we move the cut-off value to the far right, everyone who is healthy will be reported as healthy, but more diseased people will be missed (because they are wrongly labelled healthy). If we move the cut-off value to the far left, everyone who is diseased will be reported as diseased, but more healthy people will be wrongly labelled 'diseased'. At this point, we need to consider factors such as cost of screening, reliability of data and (most importantly) medical ethics. Is telling someone they have cancer when they don't as serious as missing someone who *does* have cancer?

## Strategy for values outside the range

Quite often the patient's blood test results will fall outside the reference range. As blood test results take the form of numbers and are not binary (like a broken arm), they can be viewed subjectively. It may be helpful to ask yourself the following questions:

1 How close is the value to the limits of the reference range? Consider FN, FP, TN, TP, and the mathematical limitations of reference ranges discussed above. This point is about the inherent variance in the range, person, blood sample, and so on.

2 Has the test been repeated?

3 Is the value increasing or decreasing over time?

4 Has the patient had surgery or intervention? An elevated range of inflammatory markers, such as C-reactive protein (CRP), erythrocyte sedimentation rate (ESR) and interleukin 6 (IL6) would be expected post-surgery.

5 Does the blood test fit with other 'indices' or family markers? Most tests fit into a family group (Hb, RBC and Hct). This point will be further explored in the case study in Chapter 2.

6 Is it clinically relevant? The patient may have competing pathologies. Some values will therefore be outside the range because they represent a pathology or condition that is being managed, such as chronic obstructive pulmonary disease (COPD), alcoholism or diabetes. You may be looking for a new out-of-range value or an unusually high value.

7 Will it change the patient's treatment? Before requesting the test, consider what you will do with the result and why you are requesting it.

However, you should bear in mind that the above questions should always be used in conjunction with local clinical procedures in your own healthcare setting.

# 2

# Case study: Interpreting abnormal results

There are numerous, comprehensive case study textbooks available. However, even these may not be relevant to a complex, chronic patient or caseload, as is often found in primary care. Therefore, instead of placing numerous, partly relevant case studies throughout the text, one sample case study is presented here. Based on a real patient's test results, it will help you think about general strategies when interpreting a complex, chronic patient. These strategies can be applied in any clinical setting.

The following case study will enable you to:

- consider reference ranges
- look at family indices
- explain why bloods are selected for patient management.

This is a female patient, aged 60, who is being treated for rheumatoid arthritis (RA) with the drug methotrexate. The HIGH/LOW values are just outside the reference range. The patient has been tested every four weeks for the last year. Test 1 and 2 (shown below) therefore took place four weeks apart. RA symptoms were present and the patient had no other symptoms.

## Table 2.1: Case study test results

| Test | Test 1 result | Test 2 result |
|---|---|---|
| **Full blood count (FBC)** | | |
| Platelets | NORMAL | NORMAL |
| **White cell markers** | | |
| White blood cell count (WBC) | HIGH | HIGH |
| Neutrophils | HIGH | HIGH |
| Lymphocytes | NORMAL | NORMAL |
| Monocytes | NORMAL | NORMAL |

| Basophils | NORMAL | NORMAL |
|---|---|---|
| **Red cell markers** | | |
| Haematocrit (Hct) | LOW | LOW |
| Haemoglobin (Hb) | NORMAL | NORMAL |
| Red blood cell count (RBC) | NORMAL | NORMAL |
| Mean cell volume (MCV) | NORMAL | NORMAL |
| Blast cells | NORMAL | NORMAL |
| **Inflammatory markers** | | |
| Plasma viscosity (PV) | HIGH | NORMAL |
| Erythrocyte sedimentation rate (ESR) | HIGH | NORMAL |
| C-reactive protein | HIGH | NORMAL |
| **Urea and electrolytes (U&Es), Kidney function:** | | |
| Sodium | NORMAL | NORMAL |
| Potassium | NORMAL | NORMAL |
| Urea | NORMAL | NORMAL |
| Creatinine | NORMAL | NORMAL |
| eGFR | NORMAL | NORMAL |
| **Liver function tests (LFTs)** | | |
| ALT | NORMAL | NORMAL |
| Alk Phos | NORMAL | NORMAL |
| Bilirubin | NORMAL | NORMAL |
| Albumin | NORMAL | NORMAL |
| Globulin | HIGH | NORMAL |

## Interpreting the case study results

Some of the blood test results for the patient in the case study are out of range. We will work through the following questions in order to interpret these results:

- What values are abnormal for the condition?
- What would the blood tests from a typical RA patient look like?
- Why have these blood tests been requested?

Finally, we will apply the strategy.

## What values are abnormal or typical for the condition?

An initial observation is that some conditions (like RA) can be cyclical, and the blood tests may not always match the clinical symptoms (see Test 2). Yet these false negatives could be problematic if this was a one-off blood test.

Looking at the values that are abnormal, we can make the following observations.

**The white cell count is high.** This count is raised in response to inflammation caused by an autoimmune response, some blood cancers and infection. The values observed, the duration of the condition and the presenting symptoms rule out a bacterial or viral infection. Given that red blood cell count (RBC) and platelet production is normal, a bone marrow dysfunction (leukaemia or myeloma) is unlikely. Hence these values are consistent with RA.

**The neutrophils are high**. Neutrophil numbers increase in response to sustained production of chemoattractants (which attract cells) like C-reactive protein (CRP) and TNF-alpha. CRP is raised relative to inflammation. Inflammation is cellular damage. Therefore CRP will rise in an autoimmune response through to severe burns and trauma. In practice, neutrophil increase is associated with bacterial infection, which causes inflammation and an increase in CRP. Neutrophils directly destroy the bacteria in the blood. In the case study, CRP and neutrophil values, the timeframe of the tests (one year) and presenting symptoms make a bacterial infection unlikely. The values are therefore consistent with an autoimmune response.

**The haematocrit (percentage of red blood cells in the whole blood) is low**. However, there are no symptoms of anaemia, the value is very close to the reference range 0.353 (low range 0.360) and crucially it doesn't fit with the other markers of red cell status. RBC and haemoglobin (Hb) are both normal. The value is not changing over time. A false positive is likely, and the result could be described as 'not clinically significant at this time'.

**Plasma viscosity (PV) is high**. PV is a marker of 'extra stuff' in the blood. In this case, it is raised due to increased white cells (neutrophils) and globulins (antibodies).

**Globulins are raised**. Globulins are a crude, surrogate measure of antibody production. The globulin count is raised when antibodies are produced, and antibodies are produced by B cells (a type of lymphocyte). Globulin increases in viral infections (a normal response by the lymphocytes to infection). But the case study patient's lymphocytes are normal and she has no symptoms. The globulins are raised in a myeloma (dysfunctional B cells), but again the lymphocyte count and globulin value make a diagnosis of myeloma unlikely. (A Bence Jones protein or electrophoresis band will confirm.) Globulins are often raised in an autoimmune response. Because the body makes antibodies to 'itself', this will not usually increase the lymphocyte count (as would be seen if the antibodies were being produced against a large viral infection, driving up lymphocyte number and antibody production).

## Why have these blood tests been requested?

This woman is typical of the patients encountered in practice – she has several different conditions, for which she is taking several types of medication. Looking at the long list of tests can be overwhelming and confusing. A useful strategy is to split the blood tests into a 'hierarchy of conditions' and discuss which ones require red flags (to be actioned quickly), referrals, interventions and repeat tests.

To monitor RA, the white cell count, neutrophils, PV, CRP and globulins have been requested. Any significant change in these values could indicate an additional bacterial infection. Thus, this suite of blood tests may be monitored by the secondary care specialist consultant for RA and by the primary care practitioner for additional infections.

To monitor the effects of methotrexate, two suites have been requested: LFTs, U&Es and FBC (red cell markers). Methotrexate can be toxic to some patients and the LFT panel will provide a red flag if this is the case. This also explains why the patient has a blood test every four weeks.

Methotrexate works in autoimmune conditions by restricting folate availability in the blood. Folate (folic acid) is the 'currency' the cells use to replicate (multiply) and grow (hence methotrexate's use as an anti-cancer therapy). Long-term restriction of folate can lead to macrocytic (high red cell volume) anaemia because red blood cell lifespan is only 12 weeks. To monitor this long-term predisposition to anaemia, RBC, Hct, Hb and MCV are measured regularly.

As a differential diagnosis, platelets (and RBC) are measured for possible bone marrow dysfunction, which could be masked by increased white cells in the autoimmune response.

U&Es are measured as a general marker of kidney function; and potassium is a red flag for a cardiac event. As a differential for anaemia, is any possible anaemia linked to renal insufficiency? Finally, U&Es are measured (in the case study) as a differential diagnosis for the LFTs. Some liver enzymes, like alkaline phosphatase (Alk Phos or ALP), are also found in the kidney. A raised ALP and normal U&Es can quickly indicate that the liver is the likely origin and cause for investigation.

# Applying the strategy

In the case study the value for haematocrit was out of range LOW. Using the strategy outlined above, can we interpret this value? Is it a false positive (FP)?

**1** How close is the value to the limits of the reference range?

*The value is very close to the reference range lower limit (0.353 compared to a normal value of 0.360).*

**2** Has the test been repeated?

*Yes, on several occasions the value has fallen within the reference range.*

**3** Is the value increasing or decreasing over time?

*No, it is consistently within a narrow range, which straddles the lower limit of the reference range.*

**4** Has the patient had surgery or intervention?

*Yes, the patient is on methotrexate, which is known to cause anaemia. This would help to explain a low Hct.*

**5** Does the blood test fit with other 'indices' or family markers?

*No, the red cell count (RBC), haemoglobin (Hb) and mean cell volume (MCV) are normal, even mid-range. It is unlikely that Hct will be decreased, and all red cell markers remain normal – especially in anaemia.*

**6** Is it clinically relevant?

*No, the patient is not reporting symptoms associated with anaemia. RBC and Hb are stable.*

**7** Will it change the patient's treatment?

*No, the patient should already be taking folic acid supplements.*

Given the above interpretation, even though Hct is reported as 'abnormal' the clinical team may decide not to take further action at this time. It may simply be a mathematical false positive (likely) or it may be a true positive but of little clinical relevance, in practice, to the patient. The team may decide to continue monitoring red cell markers and ask about symptoms of anaemia and folic acid compliance. Given the normal Hb, RBC and MCV, a course of iron (ferrous supplements) is unlikely to be of any benefit.

# 3

# The full blood count

The full blood count (FBC) test provides information about the cellular components of the blood. The FBC can be used in detecting anaemia, understanding inflammation and infection, and monitoring coagulation and leukaemia presentation.

The FBC result is usually made up of three components: the red cell indices, the white cell indices and the platelets. Table 3.1 (below) shows how red blood cell count (RBC), white blood cell count (WBC) and platelets alone can initially be used to stratify some indicative conditions (matched to symptoms).

## Table 3.1: Full blood count sample results

| Condition | RBC | WBC | Platelets |
|---|---|---|---|
| Anaemia | LOW | NORMAL | NORMAL |
| Infection | NORMAL | HIGH | NORMAL |
| Autoimmune conditions | NORMAL | HIGH | NORMAL |
| Leukaemia | LOW | HIGH | LOW |
| RA, methotrexate, no folate | LOW | HIGH | NORMAL |
| Aplastic anaemia, bone marrow failure | LOW | LOW | LOW |

## The red blood cell indices

These will usually be haemoglobin (Hb), haematocrit (Hct) and RBC.

Hb is the oxygen-carrying protein in red blood cells (erythrocytes) and it can be used as a marker for surgical outcome. It can also be compared to other red cell indices, such as anaemia (Hb low). In addition, it can be used as a surrogate marker of renal insufficiency (low), blood loss (low), oxygen deprivation (high) or glucose in excess (HbA1C), and in genotyping for some sickle cell conditions.

**it the right size. If the instructions have a misprint of 95 litres then more air is added and the tent will be bigger than expected.** Possible causes of this could be liver disease, pregnancy, some antibiotics, and folate and $B_{12}$ deficiency.

If folate is low, it could be due to dietary factors or a genetic defect in the enzyme (MTHFR) or some medications such as anti-cancer or epileptic drugs, or alcohol intake (◄► deranged LFTs). Alcohol can affect the stomach lining and reduce folate absorption. As red blood cells last for around 12 weeks, it would take sustained alcohol intake to change the entire RBC profile.

If $B_{12}$ is low, it could be dietary or could be due to an autoimmune pernicious anaemia (PA), which can affect the stomach lining and reduce oral $B_{12}$ absorption. A positive parietal cell and/or intrinsic factor antibody test can confirm PA. Given that oral absorption is restricted in PA, an intra-muscular $B_{12}$ injection is usually required. Failure to correct $B_{12}$ deficiency may lead to $B_{12}$ neuropathy and demyelination because $B_{12}$ is required to make the myelin sheath. If the myelin sheath is dysfunctional then nerve integrity is lost and neural and vascular retraction from the site (usually feet) will occur. ◄► Patients who are positive for parietal cell or intrinsic factor antibodies may also be positive for anti-thyroid antibodies and have low T4 (thyroxine). A thyroid function test (TFT) may therefore be appropriate.

In summary, using the MCV test from the FBC can help to differentiate between microcytic, normocytic and macrocytic anaemia.

## Anaemia of chronic disease

Some patients with long-term chronic conditions, particularly ones with an underlying inflammatory disorder such as COPD, may develop anaemia of chronic disease (ACD). In the normal red cell model, iron (Fe) is stored as ferritin. In states of low ferritin, the capacity to bind iron increases. This is called total iron binding capacity (TIBC). In a normal dietary or gastrointestinal iron-deficient anaemia, the patient will usually have a low MCV and low ferritin, but a high TIBC. In ACD, the route by which the stored iron is utilised to make red cells is compromised or broken. The cell has plenty of stored iron so it doesn't need to bind any more. Thus, in ACD serum ferritin is often high and TIBC is low. But the iron is locked in, so the cell can't use it to make red blood cells.

## Neuropathies

In addition to pernicious anaemia, $B_{12}$ neuropathy (low RBC, low $B_{12}$, high MCV, normal LFT) and diabetic and alcoholic neuropathies may co-compete in practice. Each has a different pathology.

In diabetic neuropathy (high HBA1C, normal RBC), glucose in excess binds directly to the nerve and blocks nerve impulses.

Alcoholic neuropathy (low RBC, high MCV, low folate and high LFTs) is due partly to direct poisoning of the nerve by alcohol, and by lack of nutrients caused by alcoholism ($B_{12}$ and proteins for the myelin sheath and folate). Folate has a number of roles in the body. We have discussed DNA creation, but it is also linked to clearing an amino acid called homocysteine (HCY). High levels of HCY are thought to affect vascular tone, making blood vessels stiff and reducing blood flow. This explains why poor diet and excessive alcohol intake are linked to peripheral vascular disease. Given its effect on vascular tone, high HCY is also a factor in gout, poor healing of fractures and infections, and cardiovascular disease.

Finally, the haematocrit (Hct) is often used as a confirmatory marker of RBC status. However, Hct is a crude marker, as it represents the proportion of the whole blood made up of red blood cells. This is usually 35–55% (or 0.35–0.55) and has been used historically because it is very cheap and very quick. Hct goes down in anaemia, and up in polycythaemia.

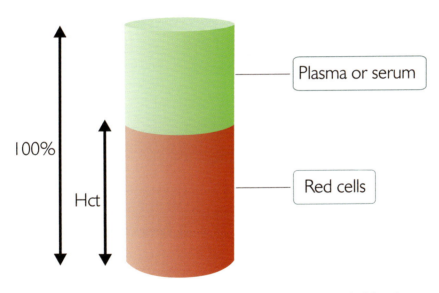

**Figure 3.2: Haematocrit as a proportion of whole blood**

## Dementia

Given that anaemia can produce some of the symptoms of dementia, it may be appropriate to screen for this, looking for low RBC or low Hb. Other exclusions include: raised inflammatory markers (erythrocyte sedimentation rate, C-reactive protein and plasma viscosity) which may indicate pulmonary vasculitis, especially with a positive ANCA test (anti-neutrophil cytoplasmic antibodies); hypothyroidism via a thyroid function test; glucose control and diabetes; and a human immunodeficiency virus (HIV) or syphilis screen.

# The white blood cell indices

Many aspects of white blood cells have already been discussed in the case study in Chapter 2. Further clinical practice examples will be explored in Chapter 5 (inflammatory markers), Chapter 6 (autoimmune conditions) and Chapters 8, 9 and 10 (chronic disease markers).

White blood cells (leukocytes) respond to, prevent and remove infection, and they are central to the inflammatory response via C-reactive protein (CRP) and TNF-alpha. There are different types of white cells, which can help identify the pathology. The white cells can either be presented as a count (a number) or as a percentage – say, 80% of the white cells are neutrophils. The percentage of white cells is called the differential or WCD.

Low WBC is a fairly rare condition (leukopenia), which is sometimes seen in patients undergoing chemotherapy. It is also found in aplastic anaemia (this is total bone marrow failure so patients will also have low RBC and low platelets), HIV (especially the T cell lymphocytes), some cases of lupus, and copper and zinc deficiency.

High WBC has three common causes, although the presenting symptoms will be different: leukaemia (usually with low RBC and low PLT), infection (look at type of white cell) and autoimmune conditions (usually raised neutrophils). ◀▶ Inflammation markers such as erythrocyte sedimentation rate (ESR), PV and CRP.

The main role of neutrophils (WCD 40–80%) is protection from bacteria and they are driven (increased) by markers of cellular damage such as CRP. They are therefore often used in autoimmune, inflammatory monitoring.

The main role of lymphocytes (10–20%) is protection from viral infection. There are two types: B cells (antibody production) and T cells (viral identification and destruction). T cells also play a role in misidentifying self-tissue in autoimmune conditions.

Monocytes (5%) infiltrate tissue in systemic bacterial tissue. Once in the tissue, they are called macrophages, and they can also incorporate low-density lipoprotein (LDL) and become a foam cell. Foam cells can then form an atherosclerotic plaque and increase cardiovascular disease risk (◀▶ cholesterol and TG concentrations and chronic disease management).

Eosinophils and basophils (5%) ensure protection from some parasites and may form a response in asthma, allergy and hypersensitivity conditions such as irritable bowel syndrome (IBS).

Blast cells (atypical, < 2%) can indicate bone marrow dysfunction. These are white cells that cannot be identified because they have been incorrectly made, and so they are often seen in leukaemia, myeloma and lymphoma.

A myeloma is a cancer of the B cell lymphocytes. Often, damaged cells aggregate in the bone (◀▶ bone pain, bone profile test and raised calcium (Ca)). The cells often produce a monoclonal globulin protein called a Bence Jones protein. The types of globulins produced by the B cells can be further assessed by means of electrophoresis, which can help differentiate between different types of myeloma and leukaemia. This gives profiles of gamma, IgG, IgM and IgD and so on. The patient will often also have raised WBC (more B cells), raised globulin (from Ab production) and raised PV due to more 'stuff' (globulins and B cells) in the blood and raised ESR.

A lymphoma is another cancer of the B cell and/or T cell lymphocyte activity, but damaged cells usually aggregate in the lymph nodes. Thus, patients are often immune-compromised, with reduced antibody production. The next step is to determine the type of lymphoma. Hodgkin's is a positive for a subset of the B cell called a Reed-Sternberg cell, which may require different treatments from non-Hodgkin's. Lymphoma patients usually have recurrent infections and are negative to Bence Jones paraprotein.

# 4

# Coagulation and deep vein thrombosis

Coagulation markers are usually used pre-operatively to prepare patients for surgery, to manage coagulation medications and to assess venous thromboembolism (VTE) risk. The usual panel will be platelets, fibrinogen, prothrombin (PT), activated partial thromboplastin time (aPTT) and international normalised ratio (INR), and D-dimer.

## Venous thromboembolism

A VTE is a clot (thrombus) in the vein, usually a deep vein thrombosis (DVT), which is dislodged (an embolism) and can move to heart, brain or lungs (pulmonary embolism or PE), with serious consequences.

VTE is most commonly caused by poor post-surgical management, or by poor lifestyle (such as a high-fat diet and sedentary habits). A VTE or DVT is diagnosed by means of a history, physical manipulation, scoring and blood tests. A combination of the ultrasound scan (US), Well's score, Homan's test and a D-dimer blood test will usually indicate a DVT diagnosis. In the UK, NICE guidelines and local operating procedures should be followed for VTE diagnosis.

The Well's score (WS) is a history-taking scoring system that takes into account active cancer, whether the patient is bedridden or has had major surgery, calf swelling in one leg, leg swollen, tender deep vein/groin, and previous DVT. The higher the Well's score, the more likely it is that a DVT may be present.

D-dimers (Dd) are fragments of a clot, which has broken down under the action of plasminogen. They are therefore indicative of a large unstable clot being resolved (DVT). This test is often used in conjunction with the Well's score[1]:

- High WS, then Dd less relevant and treatment initiated
- Medium/Low WS, negative Dd, then unlikely DVT
- Medium/Low WS, positive Dd, then usually ultrasound scan.

---

[1] These statements are examples of context and clinical advice to explain DVT, Well's score, ultrasound and D-dimer blood test. For patient management in the UK, see NICE VTE guidance.

The D-dimer test can also be used following treatment, to confirm that the clot has been fully resolved. As VTE and DVT treatment is fairly well tolerated by most patients (and in view of the complications that may result from misdiagnosis or delay), the treatment is often given on symptom presentation alone.[2] Current guidelines propose an ultrasound within four hours.

Raised platelets (thrombocythaemia) can also lead to increased risk of VTE and DVT. Raised platelets can be caused by myeloproliferative diseases such as chronic myeloid leukaemia (CML) and polycythaemia vera. These cause over-production of platelets by the bone marrow. A positive Philadelphia chromosome confirms CML.

## Coagulation monitoring

Coagulation is a clotting process that is usually initiated by tissue damage and augmented by the platelets. It has two components: intrinsic (driven by platelets) and extrinsic (driven by tissue). Both ultimately lead to fibrinogen and then to fibrin, which forms a clot complex with the platelets. (◀▶This process also produces an inflammatory response, so it makes sense also to measure white blood cell count.) This leads to an increase in erythrocyte sedimentation rate (ESR) through increased fibrinogen-sticking red blood cells.

Warfarin generally works by suppressing the liver's production of factors that induce clotting. This process is extrinsic, as it is in the liver and outside the blood. It is also relatively slow, as it takes up to five days for warfarin to work.

The usual blood test for warfarin is the international normalised ratio (INR), which essentially measures how long it takes the blood to clot in a lab, converted to an arbitrary value of 1. If, following warfarin, the INR rises to 2, the blood is therefore taking twice as long to clot. Generally, an INR greater than 4 is problematic for bleed management, and may affect decisions about micro-surgery and injection interventions.

The INR is ultimately a marker of fibrinogen production, and thus liver function (as this is where fibrinogen is made). It is also used as a surrogate marker of liver function in patients who are not on warfarin. If INR is measured in an alcoholic patient (it is quick and cheap) and the result is 7, liver dysfunction would be highly likely.

Heparin, clexane, deltaparin and low molecular weight heparin work via an intrinsic pathway, inside the blood, by directly binding to (and thus deactivating) chemicals that induce a clot. These medications will therefore work very quickly (within a few minutes) and can also be used as a prophylaxis. In view of their quick action, they are often given as a dual therapy

[2]These statements are examples of context and clinical advice to explain DVT, Well's score, ultrasound and D-dimer blood test. For patient management in the UK, see NICE VTE guidance.

with warfarin, as the latter takes a few days to work. In primary care, blood tests are less likely to be ordered for patients on these types of therapies. The test to assess these interventions is called aPTT and is usually ordered before invasive intervention.

The final group of therapies work on the platelets so they are intrinsic and can be assessed by aPTT. These include aspirin and clopidogrel. The drugs are converted in the liver into pro-drugs, which remain in production for a few days after the oral base drug has ceased. The platelets express sticky surface proteins (like a Velcro coat), which enable them to stick together and clot. This protein is called Von Willebrand's factor (VWF) and it is suppressed by the pro-drug. Once suppressed, it is likely that the platelets will have suppressed clotting ability for their lifespan of up to two weeks. Patients on high doses of such treatments may need platelet replacement to prevent bleeds – though not while the pro-drug is being made by the liver, as this will simply affect the newly transfused platelets.

Alcohol works on both intrinsic and extrinsic pathways. **Analogy: Acutely, alcohol 'gets the platelets drunk' by suppressing their VWF activity. This makes them take off their sticky coats and reduces their ability to stick together. Hence, sword fighting after drinking wine is not a good idea!** In alcoholic patients, this acute phase is augmented by liver dysfunction – the liver does not produce fibrinogen and clotting times increase significantly.

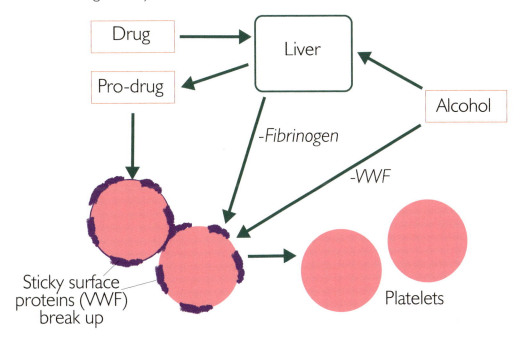

Figure 4.1: The interaction between alcohol, drugs and the liver

Finally, certain haemophilic conditions (such as an absence of VWF or of factors such as Leiden V) will also increase clotting time. In the UK, most inborn errors of metabolism and coagulation are seen in neonates. Patients with sickle cell anaemia or thalassaemia may also have a shorter red cell lifespan. This may give them a predisposition towards abnormally shaped cells, which are likely to stick together, forming a clot. The clot may then cause a painful 'crisis' and in some cases a stroke.

# 5

# Inflammatory markers

A typical inflammatory marker panel would be erythrocyte sedimentation rate (ESR), C-reactive protein (CRP) and plasma viscosity (PV). Each test tells us something different about the inflammation pathway, and some tests are more appropriate than others.

There are numerous inflammatory markers. In practice, these tests tend to be requested in two ways: either as a typical inflammatory marker panel (CRP, ESR, PV); or as a specific test, given the new interest in this area for research and drug treatments. Inflammatory markers are usually cellular signalling molecules (signal cells) or adhesion molecules (which make cells stick to the vascular wall). These adhesion molecules include tumour necrosis factor alpha (TNF alpha), interleukin-6 (IL-6), iCAM and vCAM, which are the basis of advanced drug treatments.

Inflammation is a response to cellular damage and the inflammatory markers generally rise in relation to the degree of tissue damage, particularly CRP (see the Chapter 2 case study). Cellular damage can be caused by infection (bacterial and/or viral), an autoimmune response, cancer and trauma.

An initial strategy is to map the inflammatory markers to interventions and symptoms. For example, if investigating a possible infection a few days after a hip or knee replacement, consideration should be given to the significantly raised inflammatory markers resulting from the surgery. A blood culture may be more appropriate. Although in practice an antibiotic is often prescribed, this may not be needed.

In inflammation resulting from cellular damage, there are two phases – cellular and exudative. Cellular inflammation is controlled by CRP and TNF-alpha and is the cellular response. Exudative inflammation is controlled by an enzyme called cyclo-oxygenase 2 (COX-2). This enzyme makes prostaglandins that modulate vasoconstriction and vasodilatation (the swelling response). COX-2 can be partly inhibited by aspirin and non-steroidal anti-inflammatory drugs (NSAIDS).

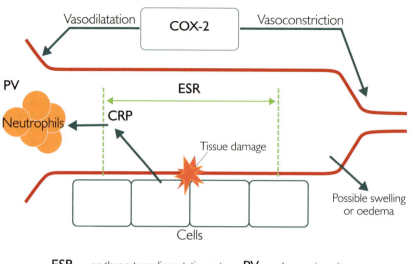

ESR – erythrocyte sedimentation rate    PV – plasma viscocity
CRP – C-reactive protein

Figure 5.1: Cellular and exudative inflammation

The tissue damage elicits a cellular signal: CRP, to recruit and increase the number of neutrophils. To aid this process, the enzyme COX-2 produces prostaglandins, which cause constriction and dilatation at the site to affect blood flow. This response may cause pain (if a nerve is part of the constricted area), swelling, oedema and redness of skin.

## Table 5.1: Inflammation analogies

**Test: C-reactive protein (CRP)**

**Analogy:**
**CRP is the 'fire alarm'.**
**The more damage there is, the more alarms will sound and the more people will ring the fire brigade.**
**Once the fire-fighters are on site, the alarms may be switched off.**

*Interpretation:*
CRP is relative to the degree of cellular damage. The more invasive the bacteria or trauma, the more CRP is produced.
If the blood test was requested post-injury, the CRP signal may be lost because the site of injury has been repaired.

**Test: Neutrophils**

**Analogy:**
**Neutrophils are the 'fire engines' that respond to CRP and cellular damage. The more damage there is, the more fire engines will be called.**
**A fire engine can also attend a fire without being called out, perhaps because the crew members have spotted a small fire on waste ground on the way back from a call (bacteria).**

*Interpretation:*
Neutrophils respond to cellular damage but can also spontaneously destroy bacteria.

---

**Test: Plasma viscosity (PV)**

**Analogy:**
**As the fire engines and debris build up in the surrounding streets, the pressure in the area will increase. The more fire engines (neutrophils) and news reporters (bacteria, for example) there are, the more blocked the street will become.**
**Even after the fire alarm (CRP) has been switched off, the engines may stay at the site for a while. Neutrophils have a lifespan of two weeks so PV may be elevated after the initial CRP value.**

*Interpretation:*
PV is a crude marker of material in the blood that increases pressure and 'thickness' or viscosity. The more cells and bacteria there are, the higher the PV.
PV can be useful to show that tissue injury occurred in the absence of a raised CRP.

---

**Test: Erythrocyte sedimentation rate (ESR)**

**Analogy:**
**Following a large fire, structural reinforcement is required. ESR indicates the amount of clotting around the damage site.**

*Interpretation:*
In some autoimmune conditions that have relatively small amounts of tissue damage, such as rheumatoid arthritis (RA), ESR may be requested on a six-monthly basis because the damage is too small to affect the ESR.

**Test: White blood cell count (WBC)**

**Analogy:**
**The white cells are the 'emergency vehicles' (police cars and fire engines). As more fire engines (neutrophils) take to the street, the number of emergency vehicles on the roads increases. The WBC is the total number of white cells in circulation.**

*Interpretation:*
WBC reflects inflammation. ◄► CRP, PV, ESR and white cell type. Increased neutrophils are likely to indicate a bacterial infection or an autoimmune response. Raised lymphocytes are likely to be due to viral infection.

## Erythrocyte sedimentation rate

The erythrocyte sedimentation rate (ESR) is 'how far red cells (erythrocytes) fall (sediment) in a tube, in an hour'. As the tissue is damaged, fibrinogen is released. Fibrinogen 'sticks' red cells together, making them heavy, so they fall further in the test. A high ESR means that more red cells are stuck together by fibrinogen, which results in more cell/tissue damage. ESR is usually raised in inflammation, but it can take time for this 'sticking process' to occur and indeed be removed. ESR is therefore not as quick to respond to damage as CRP. In some cases, ESR will rise in anaemia (independently of fibrinogen and inflammation). Large, macrocytic red blood cells will fall more quickly than small or normal-size ones.

**Analogy: If you went to the top of a tall building and dropped three footballs (red cells), timing how long they took to fall, that would be a normal ESR. If you repeated this exercise, but placed the footballs in a heavy sack (fibrinogen resulting from inflammation), the balls would fall faster. However, as discussed earlier, ESR can also be independent of inflammation. If you repeated the demonstration, but dropped a large medicine ball (a macrocytic red blood cell) instead of three footballs, the large ball would fall faster. In other words, ESR can also be raised in macrocytic anaemia. You could cross-check ESR with mean cell volume (MCV) to find out the size of the red cells.**

# Plasma viscosity

Plasma viscosity (PV) is a measure of pressure *in* the blood (not blood pressure). It is measured in mPascals, a unit of pressure. PV is a surrogate marker of material that is not expected to be in the blood. As more white cells, bacteria, antibodies, red cells, in fact any material, build up in the blood, the pressure will rise and so will PV. It's often described as 'thick blood' because more material is present.

**Analogy: Visualise a glass filled with water, and imagine stirring it with a spoon. The amount of pressure or power needed to stir the water is a normal PV. If you add a handful of marbles to the glass, it will be harder to stir because more pressure will be needed. Now imagine the glass is inside a box so you can't see what is causing it to get harder to stir. It could be marbles (red blood cells), but it could also be stones (white blood cells) or woollen fibres (antibodies) or even sand (bacteria). Hence, an increased PV demonstrates an increase in pressure within the blood. But to determine the cause you'll need to cross-check with other tests such as full blood count (FBC), looking at WBC, RBC and so on.**

PV is mainly used to understand inflammation. It's used in autoimmune conditions because it can indicate that additional antibodies and white cells are present, thickening or increasing pressure in the blood. PV can also be useful for monitoring against a baseline over time. However, it has limitations in that it is not specific to one disease and is therefore a crude global marker.

# CRP

C-reactive protein (CRP) is a molecule that attracts and induces production of white blood cells (usually neutrophils), following inflammation. CRP is a marker for inflammation and infection and it can be used in autoimmune conditions because it can represent cellular signalling. CRP is also being used for chronic disease surveillance, as it is sensitive enough to represent vascular damage (raised CRP) and liver disease (low CRP). However, in some settings it can be expensive. Also, the signal can be lost as CRP is cleared, whilst ESR and PV may remain high for some time after the initial response.

The following analogy offers a strategy to assist in interpreting a complex and dynamic process.

**Analogy: CRP is the fire alarm that goes off in the building, attracting fire engines (neutrophils/WBC) and causing a traffic jam in the street (PV). The structural support (fibrinogen scaffold) around the building is ESR. It's unlikely that a small fire, as in the specific connective tissue damage caused by rheumatoid arthritis, will result in the entire building needing scaffolding. ESR is therefore only requested periodically, usually every six months. However, following major surgery or a large muscle trauma, ESR would be required.**

## Anti-inflammatory treatments

Anti-inflammatory treatments work along the pathways shown in Figure 6.1 (see page 37). Anti-TNF alpha treatments suppress the initial chemoattractant; drugs like methotrexate work by suppressing the neutrophil recruitment and replication (it was originally an anti-cancer cell proliferation drug); and drugs like aspirin and NSAIDS work to inhibit COX-2 and relieve the vasoconstriction.

To summarise, ESR represents tissue repair post-injury (fibrinogen), PV reflects components in the blood due to inflammation (more WBC, more antibodies), and CRP represents the tissue signalling in response to cellular damage.

# Autoimmune conditions

In an autoimmune disease, our white cells destroy our own cells. The most common reason for this is incorrect cellular signalling, when the cell expresses a 'self-antigen'. Most autoimmune diagnostic tests are based on detecting the presence of self-antigen or auto-antibodies.

## Normal response to viral infection

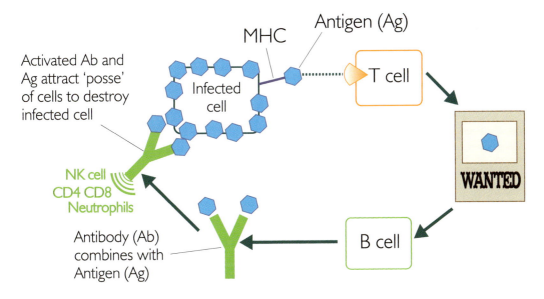

Figure 6.1: A normal response to a viral infection

In Figure 6.1, the virus uses the internal machinery of the cell to replicate itself. It then bursts the cell and infects an adjacent cell. Because the virus is small (compared to bacteria), the cell needs to make the white cells aware that it has been infected.

**Analogy: The virus inside the infected cell is too small to be detected by the white cells. The infected cell spreads the news of the infection to the white**

**cells by taking a small part of the virus, called an antigen (Ag), and 'placing it on a stick' outside the cell. This stick is called major histocompatibly complex (MHC). The T cell (a type of lymphocyte) then acts like a camera and takes a picture of the MHC/Ag. Having taken the photo, the T cell uses it to make a 'Wanted poster' of the MHC/Ag 'villain' and shows the poster to the B cell (a type of lymphocyte). The B cell makes antibodies (Ab) specifically designed to counteract the Ag, and the tailor-made Ab binds itself to the Ag. Once bound, a signal is activated and this attracts a 'posse' of neutrophils, natural killer cells and CD4/CD8 cytotoxic T cells to destroy the cell hosting the villainous virus.**

The process of destroying the virus usually causes cellular damage. It increases C-reactive protein (CRP), produces more neutrophils and plasma viscosity (PV), and raises WBC (white cell or lymphocyte count). For example, human immunodeficiency virus (HIV) destroys the T cells and so the lymphocyte count may actually go down. With the T cell 'camera' not working, AIDS patients may be susceptible to otherwise benign viral infections.

This can also be seen when diagnosing viral hepatitis. For example, the presence of hepatitis B surface antigen (HepBsAg) may indicate a current infection. Likewise, the presence of HepB Ab will suggest a live infection (if HepBsAg is also present), a successful vaccination, or the presence of the disease in the past (as the B cells have made a specific Ab for HepB). There is also a new, rapid technique available that measures the DNA or RNA of the HepB virus directly in the cell. This is helpful in children or acute cases, as it may otherwise take a few days or even months for the patient to produce enough Ag or Ab to be measured (◀▶ the hepatitis virus that damages the hepatocyte, which often increases the liver enzyme ALT).

## Autoimmune basics

In autoimmune conditions, there is *no* viral infection. But for some reason (which is still unclear at present), a part of the cell's own protein is placed 'on the stick'. This causes the same chain of events, which leads to the production of a specific antibody. Broadly, for rheumatoid arthritis this Ab is rheumatoid factor (RF); for ankylosing spondylitis (AS) it is HLAb27; for pernicious anaemia it is parietal cell Ab or intrinsic factor Ab; and for systemic lupus erythematosus (SLE) it is anti-nucleic antibody (ANA).

There are hundreds of possible Ab tests, usually undertaken in secondary care by a consultant. If the Ab is present then the patient is called 'seropositive'; if it is not present then the patient is labelled 'seronegative'. For most Ab tests, about 80% of people with the symptoms are seropositive, leaving 20% seronegative. For these seronegative patients, we could undertake more Ab tests. However, in practice it's more likely that their symptoms will be treated as if they were positive and the effects reviewed. The reason for the existence of symptoms in seronegative patients is unclear.

As discussed in the case study in Chapter 2, autoimmune patients may have blood tests to consider the autoimmune diagnosis (RF), white cell and inflammation response to the condition (WBC, neutrophils, CRP, PV) and any effects of treatments or interventions (RBC, MCV, folate, LFTs and U&Es).

There are also antibodies, called anti-neutrophil cytoplasmic antibodies (ANCA), which 'attack' and then change the role of neutrophils. They are commonly associated with vasculitis, which is the inflammatic destruction of the vasculature; cANCA is associated with granulomatosis with polyangiitis (Wegener's) affecting lungs and kidney; whilst pANCA is associated with glomerular nephritis (◀▶ U&Es). Both types can be associated with ankylosing spondylitis (AS).

Clinical symptoms will drive some of the decision-making in terms of requesting and interpreting autoimmune blood tests. For example, a patient with AS will usually have a different presentation from one with RA. As discussed in Chapter 2, these patients may already have outlying values for WBC, CRP and PV because of their underlying condition. As the condition flares, these changes may be significant but nevertheless clinically expected given the condition. However, we still need to be aware that another new condition (such as a bacterial infection) could also modulate WBC, CRP and PV, so we should question baseline changes and symptoms.

## Typical autoimmune profiles

A typical systemic lupus erythematosus (SLE) blood profile could be that about 95% of patients with SLE have a positive ANA. SLE is often seen with thrombocytopenia (low platelets) and high levels of anti-single-stranded DNA Ab (a type of antibody usually found in these conditions, usually requested by a consultant).

A typical RA blood profile could be that about 80% of patients are positive for RF and negative for HLAb27. This often occurs with raised neutrophils and WBC, raised CRP, raised PV and raised globulin.

A typical AS blood profile could be that about 80% of patients are positive for HLAb27 and negative for RF. If a patient is HLAb27 negative then we could consider two new genetic tests: Type 1 tumour necrosis factor receptor shedding aminopeptidase regulator (ARTS1) and interleukin 23 receptor (IL23R). This often occurs with raised neutrophils, WBC, CRP and erythrocyte sedimentation rate (ESR).

Polymyalgia rheumatica (PMR) means 'pain in many muscles' and is thought to be mainly due to inflammation of the muscle's vascular system. A typical PMR blood profile could be raised ESR and CRP. These patients are usually negative to rheumatoid factor (RF) but positive to HLAb27, and some have elevated platelets and low RBC (although the reason is unclear). If the patient is on certain types of statins, measuring total creatine kinase (CK) may help identify muscle damage. CK is a muscle enzyme and its value in the blood increases in relation to muscle damage. It is thought that some statins can induce muscle damage and cause pain.

Polymyositis is the presentation of muscle antigen as foreign material. A typical blood profile could be positive for ANA and then positive for the Anti Jo subset (a type of antibody usually found in these conditions). These patients could also have raised serum creatinine kinase (CK), and usually raised CRP, PV and ESR.

Reactive arthritis is often linked to an underlying viral or bacterial infection that has induced an immune response and is not subsequently 'switched off'. A typical blood profile could be positive for HLAb27 and negative for RF, with raised CRP and ESR.

Psoriatic arthritis (PA) causes connective and musculo-skeletal damage, which is usually linked to prolonged psoriasis. Psoriasis is the autoimmune destruction of the skin, and a typical PA profile could be negative for RF but positive for HLAb27, with raised CRP and ESR.

# 7

# Transfusion testing

As blood transfusion involves the transfer of either whole blood or specific blood products between patients, certain screening tests need to be conducted. It may also be appropriate to screen patients' blood to ascertain their blood group or rhesus (Rh) status in case they subsequently require an intervention. Haematology and biochemistry are closely related areas so blood samples for transfusion or blood products might be requested at the same time. Typical tests would include ABO group and Rh type, blood group antibodies, syphilis, HIV and HepB.

The ABO blood group is determined by surface antigens and corresponding antibodies. In A group, the red cell has A antigens and thus anti-B antibodies in the plasma, as the presence of a red blood cell with a B antigen would suggest a foreign or exogenous source. In B group, the red cell has B surface antigens and thus anti-A antibodies in the plasma. For this reason, A blood cannot usually be given to B blood patients. In AB blood group, the red cell has both A and B surface antigens and therefore has *no* antibodies in the blood. Hence, a person with AB can usually receive any blood group. In O blood group, the red cell has *no* surface antigens but usually has both A and B antibodies. Hence, O can usually be given to all groups. As the plasma and red cells contain opposing antigens and antibodies, plasma compatibility is usually the opposite of red cell compatibility.

Rh type denotes the presence or absence of a D antigen, with Rhesus positive (Rh+) having the D antigen present. The Rh type is identified in addition to the antigen status of the red blood cell, for example, O- or AB+. People who are Rhesus negative (Rh-) can usually receive blood from matched ABO Rh- type, whereas Rh+ patients can usually receive either Rh- or Rh+ type.

Whole blood products can also be separated into their component parts: packed red cells from which most of the liquid component (plasma) has been removed; plasma; platelets; and fresh frozen plasma (FFP), plasma that is rapidly frozen which helps to retain key clotting factors.

Hepatitis screening for HepB (HBV) is usually done by checking for the HBsAg or HBcAb, the former being the surface antigen and the latter being the antibody. Some departments may offer the nucleic acid test, which determines the presence of HepB viral RNA. If the patient has an active infection then they are likely to have the antigen and/or the RNA, as well as the antibody (which may take a few weeks to develop). Hepatitis C (HBC) is usually tested by the presence of the HBC antibody.

**Analogy: Thinking about the A blood group in the ABO system, the white cells are your 'protective army' who will destroy foreign invaders. If you clearly mark *your* red blood cells with a *red* flag (A Ag), your army will NOT destroy cells with a red flag. But it WILL destroy cells with a blue flag, using its special anti-blue flag rockets (the anti-B Ab). You can therefore give your blood to other people with red-flagged cells, but not to people with anti-red flag rockets. AB people have red cells with BOTH red and blue flags, so they have NO anti-red or anti-blue rockets and can receive any type of red cell. In O group blood, the red cell has NO flags. O group blood can therefore be given to people in any group, even if they have anti-red or or anti-blue flag rockets. People with O blood can therefore usually only receive type O blood. Hence, type O blood is often referred to as 'universal donor', while type AB blood is a 'universal receiver'.**

# 8

# Chronic disease markers: Diabetes

In practice, especially in primary care, patients usually present with one (or both) of the two major types of diabetes: diabetes insipidus (DI) and diabetes mellitus (DM), with resulting polyuria and dehydration.

## Diabetes insipidus

Diabetes insipidus is not usually linked to excessive glucose but instead to deficient control of anti-diuretic hormones that control urine output. Investigations to help differentiate DM from DI include: raised glucose and HBa1C, indicating DM; raised Na, suggesting DM and DI; and low vasopressin (antidiuretic hormone (ADH) indicating DI). In both types of diabetes, kidney function may be affected so you should also consider measuring U&Es.

DI has three causes: neurogenic (no vasopressin production in the brain); nephrogenic (kidney does not respond to vasopressin); and dipsogenic (inappropriate thirst mechanism triggered by the hypothalamus, which incorrectly suppresses vasopressin). To differentiate, a desmopressin fluid intake test may be conducted. Alternatively, renal function can be assessed by U&Es (raised Na and urea, and decreased estimated glomerular filtration rate or eGFR), or a thyroid function test can be performed to exclude a tumour (abnormally high or low levels of TRH, TSH and T4). See Chapter 11 on thyroid function tests.

## Diabetes mellitus

Diabetes mellitus is a generic name for poor control of glucose. Patients with DM have high levels of glucose (hyperglycaemia) due to a poor insulin response. The main presenting symptom in primary care is polyuria due to osmotic diuresis. This is caused by excessive glucose in the kidney, which cannot be reabsorbed. Osmotic pressure is increased within the tubule, which transiently retains water within the lumen, thus increasing urine output. This subsequently leads to dehydration (polydipsia). There are two main types of DM: Type 1, in which no insulin is produced; and Type 2, in which insulin is not effectively recognised by cell receptors.

Glucose is a type of sugar (a carbohydrate) and provides the primary source of energy in the body, especially in the brain, which is why it needs to be stored effectively. Free glucose, in the blood, lasts a few hours before we become hungry; and stores of glucose last about 16 to 24 hours before hypoglycaemia and confusion occur. Glucose is also highly reactive. It will bind readily to DNA and protein, causing most of the symptoms of diabetes, such as neuropathy, retinopathy and erectile dysfunction. Polyuria is partly caused by destruction of the glomeruli in the kidney and partly because glucose also drives water balance, and thus polydipsia. Hence, there is a vital need to clear excess glucose.

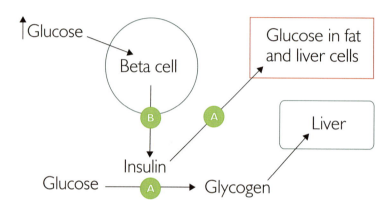

A Type 2: Unable to respond to insulin
B Type 1: Unable to make insulin

**Figure 8.1: Flow diagram of insulin-mediated storage of glucose as glycogen**

Glucose causes insulin to be released from beta cells in the pancreas. Insulin converts glucose to glycogen (in a process called glycogenesis), and the glycogen is subsequently stored in the liver. Failure to recognise glucose or make insulin will lead to glucose in excess. Glucose levels can therefore, in a normal state, be affected by stress, pancreatitis and liver damage (◀▶ adrenaline, amylase (raised in pancreatitis) and LFTs, especially following trauma or in patients with poor liver function).

## Diabetic complications

Most of the complications in diabetes are caused by excess glucose binding to, and then interfering with the actions of, specialised cells and proteins.

There is raised cardiovascular risk caused by excess glucose binding to the vascular wall. This increases stiffness and oxidises any excess low-density lipoprotein (LDL), which – under the action of macrophages – becomes foam cells and forms atherosclerotic plaques. The glucose also binds directly to the cardiac muscle and nerve endings.

In diabetic neuropathies, the excess glucose binds directly to the nerve cells and suppresses nerve conductivity, inducing vascular and neural retraction from the site. The reduction in vascular flow and integrity leads to more incidents of infection because the white cells are less able to reach the affected site. This is also why antibiotic therapies may take longer to work. This is particularly true in sites with poor circulation such as hands and feet, where neuropathies are most commonly observed in primary care.

In diabetic retinopathy and other vision symptoms, the excess glucose binds directly to the retinal cells and changes their structure. This causes a change in opacity and function, leading to blurred vision and in some cases eventual loss of sight.

In diabetic renal impairment, the excess glucose binds directly to the glomerulus and nephrons, suppressing performance. This often reduces eGFR and increases the already dysfunctional Na levels caused by polyuria and polydipsia.

Diabetic ketoacidosis occurs when fatty acids are utilised for energy, given the poor control of glucose. This produces ketones, which are acidic and affect the blood pH. Investigations should include high blood glucose, presence of ketone bodies, high blood pH, U&E due to renal dysfunction due to continued dehydration, amylase to rule out pancreatitis, and full blood count (FBC) and C-reactive protein (CRP) to rule out infection.

## Measuring glucose, and diagnosing and treating diabetes

Glucose levels can be measured in numerous ways, shown A to D in Figure 8.2 (below).

Random blood glucose (A) assesses the patient's ability at a random point to have glucose under control. This is usually used in patients already diagnosed with diabetes, who are managing insulin loads or diet interventions. The random blood glucose can produce false positive values (B), particularly following a meal, especially if the meal is high in sugar. This false positive would return to normal values under the action of insulin over a few hours. Fasted blood glucose (B1) may therefore be requested to remove the chance of a high result being due to a meal.

The oral glucose tolerance test (C) measures the insulin response following a glucose load. The patient attends having fasted and a blood sample is taken (time = 0 min). The patient is then given a glucose load, usually as a drink, which should induce an insulin response. They then wait in a low exercise capacity, for two hours, for the action of biphasic insulin to be effective. Then a second blood test is taken (time = 120 min). Glucose is measured and compared in both samples; they should be within the reference range in normal patients. In glucose intolerant or diabetic patients, the 120-minute sample will have glucose outside the reference range (C1), highlighting a lack of insulin efficacy.

HbA1c is a type of haemoglobin (HbA) with glucose attached to it (D). Haemoglobin is the oxygen-carrying protein in red blood cells and it becomes irreversibly glycosylated when glucose is in excess. It is therefore a useful long-term marker of diabetes, because the red blood cell has a lifespan of 12 weeks. There are two ways to express HbA1c – either as a percentage or as a concentration. The DCCT percentage values refer to what percentage of total Hb is HbA1c. A value higher than 7% usually indicates glucose intolerance. The ICCT mmol/mol value refers to measuring the amount of HbA1c directly as a concentration. A value higher than 53 mmol/mol usually reflects glucose intolerance.

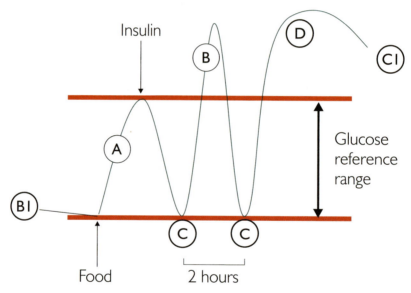

Figure 8.2: Measuring glucose levels

Drugs like metformin (a biguanide class) work by inhibiting hepatic glucose production. This decreases glucose uptake in the gut and increases insulin-sensitive receptors, which increases cellular glucose uptake. Successful treatment with metformin should reduce excess glucose and may also reduce LDL and coronary heart disease risk.

Drugs like exenatide (byetta) work by increasing pancreatic insulin, suppressing glucose transit across the gut and suppressing glucagon (a hormone released to suppress insulin activity via negative feedback).

# Chronic disease markers: Cholesterol

The risk of developing cardiovascular disease (CVD) can be measured using a variety of tests within the UK NHS Quality and Outcomes Framework (QOF) – for example, the percentage of patients with coronary heart disease (CHD) whose last measured total cholesterol (measured in the previous 15 months) is 5mmol/l or less.

Wider lifestyle choices could also be addressed with full blood count (FBC), liver function tests (LFTs) and cholesterol measures. Red blood cell count (RBC) may be increased in response to tissue hypoxia caused by smoking (polycythaemia), which may elevate plasma viscosity (PV) and increase clot risk. The presence of plasma cotinine can be used as a marker of nicotine exposure in an active smoker. Homocysteine is an amino acid that causes arterial stiffness, and is present in folate deficiency (often caused by the poor diet seen in smokers and alcoholics). Other tests would include an increased gamma-glutamyl transferase (GGT), which would also suggest alcohol intake (see LFTs, chapter 14). Total cholesterol should be checked as a CHD marker, using HbA1c or fasting glucose to address any underlying diabetes. Finally, there may be a link to hypothyroidism, which should be investigated with a thyroid function test. A genetic condition called familial hypercholesterolaemia should also be checked as appropriate.

## 'Good' and 'bad' cholesterol

Cholesterol has several functions: development of cell membranes; production of bile (which makes fats soluble and absorbs vitamins); and production of vitamin D and steroids (cortisol and aldosterone) and sex hormones (progesterone, oestrogen and testosterone). Cortisol releases glucose in response to stress, and aldosterone increases blood pressure. These are evolutionary fight-or-flight mechanisms, *but* high stress, glucose and high blood pressure are all lifestyle risks in CVD.

As cholesterol is fat-soluble and is needed by various cells, it is transported in the water-based blood by chylomicrons. 'Bad' low-density lipoprotein (LDL) and 'good' high-density lipoprotein (HDL) are types of chylomicrons.

**Analogy: LDL is like a ferry that delivers cholesterol (logs to build things with) from the liver (mainland) to the cell (an island). HDL is another ferry that takes the excess cholesterol (spare logs) back to the mainland to be destroyed. If the diet is high in cholesterol, more log-laden ferries leave for the island. But there isn't always a corresponding increase in ferries to remove the excess cholesterol. Over time, the LDL logs can therefore build up on the island. Macrophages (white cells) then invade the island, thinking there is a problem. The white cells set fire to the log pile, triggering an immune response, which leads to clotting. This significant change in cellular architecture is supported by clotting and keratinisation of the area, creating an atherosclerotic plaque. If the plaque becomes dislodged, a cardiac event may occur. Cholesterol may also lead to plaque formation in cardiac wall structures (◀▶ inflammation, FBC and the use of C-reactive protein (CRP) as a CVD risk predictor).**

## Cardiovascular risk

Total cholesterol is usually measured with the patient having fasted. It is a complex equation, which takes into account LDL cholesterol, HDL cholesterol and triglycerides. The National Institute for Health and Clinical Excellence (NICE) and Department of Health cholesterol guidelines specify a normal/healthy threshold of total cholesterol less than 5.0mmol/l and LDL cholesterol less than 3.0mmol/l.

HDL transports cholesterol from the arterial wall and blood to the liver (to be excreted) and adrenal glands (to be used to make cortisol). In this way, HDL helps to reduce cholesterol levels and CHD risk and may also modulate CVD risk by directly inhibiting the LDL-induced inflammation and platelet aggregation in the vasculature.

## Triglycerides

Triglycerides (TGs) are the fat equivalent of glycogen. They are stored fat molecules. Some TGs are transported in the blood between adipose tissue and muscle and therefore reflect a high-fat diet. There is a relationship between high TGs and low HDL, although the reasons why a high TG level is a risk factor for CVD are not fully understood. One hypothesis is that the 'type of fat' (such as omega 3) being incorporated into the vascular wall may be more (or less) susceptible to being oxidised. This may lead to the vascular wall becoming more (or less) structurally 'stiff'. If the vascular wall becomes less able to flex, this increases CHD risk.

# Cholesterol treatments

Statins reduce cholesterol/LDL production in the liver by partly suppressing the enzymes HMG-CoA reductase and Acetyl-CoA. **Analogy: These enzymes help to load the logs onto the ferry in the liver in order to deliver the cholesterol to the vascular walls.** By suppressing this activity, the cholesterol delivery (total cholesterol in the blood) is reduced. A side effect in some patients is the separate induction of muscle destruction, leading to muscle pain. Some practices may simply choose to change the statins, but in some cases it may be appropriate to measure muscle damage. A helpful test for this is total creatine kinase (CK). Muscle pain with creatine kinase (CK) levels more than ten times the upper limit of normal (ULN) may indicate clinically important myositis and rhabdomyolysis. If pain continues following statin withdrawal, an additional pathology may be present.

Cholesterol is usually used as a predictor of CHD. Another predictive cardiac marker is b-type natriuretic peptide (BNP). An increase in BNP correlates with increased cardiac wall load and dysfunction.

Following a cardiac event, endogenous cardiac muscle proteins or enzymes (due to the muscle damage) are present in the blood. CKmb is a type of creatine kinase found in heart tissue, which is released into the blood following cardiac damage, making it a useful indicator of a cardiac event. CK muscle brain (CKmb) rises after three hours, and myoglobin rises after seven hours. Aspartate aminotransferase (AST) may rise after two days. (AST is a liver enzyme, but it is also found in the heart – ◀▶ normal other LFT values.)

Troponins peak after seven hours and remain elevated for up to seven days. Troponins are muscle structure (contraction) proteins, which are released into the blood after muscle damage. Troponin I and C are markers of cardiac muscle damage, which is commonly used to differentiate between an angina and a myocardial infarction (MI). MI often results in significant troponin I release compared to angina, although care is needed when making a final interpretation, as some non-myocardial events (like tachycardia) can raise troponins. Patients with chronic obstructive pulmonary disease (COPD) may also have increased levels of troponins, given the ischemic and hypoxic nature of the disorder.

# 10

# Chronic disease markers:
## Chronic obstructive pulmonary disease and acid base

Chronic obstructive pulmonary disorder (COPD) is a narrowing of the airways, leading to poor lung function and severe airflow obstruction (low $FEV_1$). The cause of COPD is not clear, although there are several contributing factors such as smoking, exposure to workplace dust and particulates, air pollution and genetic factors (in about 2% of cases). It can also partly result from an autoimmune condition following prolonged inflammation, as seen in other autoimmune conditions.

Patients with COPD may be more susceptible to upper and lower pulmonary infections – hence the importance of vaccinations. White blood cell count (WBC) may be a helpful marker for infection, as would the presence of a functional antibody (Ab) following vaccination.

Given the restriction in oxygen caused by COPD, the patient may develop polycythaemia with a raised red blood cell count (RBC), especially if they also smoke. However, in practice, in an elderly patient, the hypoxia-induced production of erythropoietin (EPO) may be mitigated by poor renal function (with an estimated glomerular filtration rate <60) and raised RBC may not occur, as EPO is made by the kidney.

In addition, tuberculosis may need to be excluded in COPD patients. It may also be appropriate to screen for alpha-1-antitrypsin, which provides important protection from attack by white cells. White cells, particularly neutrophils, use potent enzymes to destroy bacteria. To protect our own cells from attack, we make alpha-1-antitrypsin, which can block or inhibit these enzymes. In some autoimmune conditions and COPD, the patient may have a deficiency or lack of alpha-1-antitrypsin and the raised neutrophils can therefore cause more damage.

## Acid base measures

Acid base measures are helpful in COPD patients, as well as in those with diabetes or drug overdose and those taking proton pump inhibitors. Acid and alkaline conditions are determined by the concentration of H ions (protons). A high $H^+$ concentration is a low acid pH, and a low $H^+$ concentration is a high alkaline pH. Most enzymes work within a narrow range of pH (around 7.4) to control these two systems, metabolic and respiratory, using the kidney and lungs respectively to ensure that this pH is maintained. Changes in $H^+$ concentrations are controlled by buffers.

The equation

$$H^+ + HCO_3^- \text{ (metabolic)} \leftrightarrows CO_2 + H_2O \text{ (respiratory)}$$

is used to describe the bicarbonate ($HCO_3$) buffer system. Thus, if the pH rises (more $H^+$), this moves the equation to the right, producing more $CO_2$, which is cleared by a subsequent increase in ventilation. Equally, a poor ventilation rate will increase $CO_2$ and move the equation to the left and increase pH. This is why COPD patients often have respiratory acidosis.

These compensatory mechanisms also function within a particular timespan. Physiological buffers, such as the bicarbonate–carbonic acid buffering system, work immediately. Pulmonary compensation occurs next, within a few minutes. Finally, about six hours after sustained acidosis or alkalosis, renal compensation occurs. In certain patients, bone can also be used as a last resort, as it contains high levels of bicarbonates, although this disrupts bone density. Therefore patients with COPD, renal dysfunction (chronic kidney disease) and bone dysfunction (osteoporosis) may have a very limited buffering capacity and will need to be carefully assessed.

## Acid base derangements

The most common acid base derangements are metabolic acidosis, metabolic alkalosis, respiratory acidosis and respiratory alkalosis.

In metabolic acidosis, the pH is low, meaning high $H^+$ load. Causes of metabolic acidosis include lactic acidosis, diabetic ketoacidosis (ketone bodies are produced from fat, which are acidic), and loss of bicarbonate through severe diarrhoea or bicarbonate wasting through the kidneys or gastrointestinal (GI) tract. This is metabolic, partly because cells are producing excess acid and partly because the kidney attempts to clear $H^+$. $H^+$ in excess can move into the cells and cause $K^+$ to be shunted out, leading to hyperkalaemia and a possible coronary heart disease event.

As $HCO_3^-$ increases (usually as the result of excessive loss of metabolic acids), metabolic alkalosis occurs. Causes of metabolic alkalosis include Cushing's syndrome, some diuretics, secretory adenoma of the colon, and exogenous steroids.

Respiratory acidosis (pH <7.35, $PaCO_2$ >45 mm Hg) reflects alveolar hypoventilation. Given that the renal control of $HCO_3^-$ is tightly controlled, large and prolonged changes of $PaCO_2$ are required to increase pH. As discussed, this is usually seen in primary care as COPD, and in acute care as brainstem injury from acute ingestion of opioids. Supportive $O_2$ treatments may be used, or in acute cases of overdose corrective therapies like intravenous naloxone may be considered.

Respiratory alkalosis usually occurs as a result of hyperventilation, often caused by mechanical over-ventilation, hepatic disease, 'panic attacks', pregnancy and septicaemia. Treatments are usually corrective, such as controlling breathing. However, the patient should be monitored to prevent subsequent metabolic acidosis.

## Table 10.1: Sample acid base results

| pH | $pCO_2$ | $HCO_3^-$ | Interpretation | Example |
|----|---------|-----------|----------------|---------|
| HIGH | LOW | NORMAL | Respiratory alkalosis | Hyperventilation |
| LOW | HIGH | NORMAL | Respiratory acidosis | COPD |
| HIGH | NORMAL | HIGH | Metabolic alkalosis (MAL) | Cushing's, Diuretics |
| LOW | NORMAL | LOW | Metabolic acidosis (MAC) | Diabetic ketoacidosis |

It is also possible to have a mixed acid base. For example, a patient who has lactic acidosis (metabolic) and COPD (respiratory) might have the following results: pH 7.12, $CO_2$ 55, $HCO_3^-$ 14, and so on.

# 11

# Thyroid function

The thyroid is a gland in the neck, which produces thyroxine, which ultimately modulates cellular energy expenditure. A thyroid function test (TFT) can be complex to interpret but most hospital departments will be able to provide detailed interpretations. A TFT has three main purposes: to diagnose problems with the thyroid (and pituitary/hypothalamus axis); to differentiate from another condition (such as pernicious anaemia, which also raises anti-thyroid antibodies); and to monitor the titration of thyroxine (T4) treatment.

In simple terms, environmental factors such as light and heat, signals from dietary status, and stress and depression send information to the hypothalamus, which produces thyrotropin-releasing hormone (TRH). TRH acts on the pituitary gland to produce thyroid-stimulating hormone or thyrotropin (TSH), which elicits thyroxine (T4) from the thyroid gland. Elevated levels of T4 can act as a negative feedback to switch off TRH production. In clinical practice, T4 will be measured if TSH is out of range.

## T3

T3 is produced from T4 and is a more biologically active thyroid hormone. In practice, since T3 is derived from T4, T4 is usually used to monitor thyroid function. However T3 can be requested if the TFT values are deranged, and further investigation is needed. T3 is helpful in the early diagnosis of hyperthyroidism (see below), as T3 rises before T4. The main uses of T3 are to monitor T3 therapy and to address hyperthyroidism in a patient with a low TSH. Remember, hyperthyroidism should usually have a high TSH. A low TSH could therefore indicate a non-thyroidal illness (NTI). NTI is usually seen in acute conditions, such as diabetic keto-acidosis, after an MI, in severe starvation and in critical patients in the intensive therapy unit (ITU). It is thought to be due to a dysfunctional thyroid pituitary hypothalamus feedback loop (see Figure 11.1 below).

**Analogy: Both T3 and T4 are usually transported by chaperone proteins like albumin. They are like young girls from wealthy Victorian families, who**

**could not travel without an elderly female companion. 'Free' T4 and T3 are like Victorian urchins from poor families, who were free to roam the streets without any chaperones. They are not bound to transporting proteins and are therefore biologically active.**

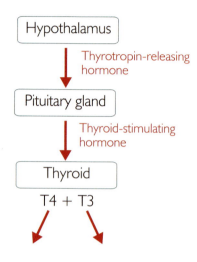

Figure 11.1: Thyroid hormones

## Hyperthyroidism

Hyperthyroidism is raised T4, leading to increased metabolic rate (often with a goitre), agitation and weight loss. Most cases are primary Grave's autoimmune, although a rare secondary form caused by a tumour of the pituitary overproducing TSH also exists. It is often treated with anti-thyroid drugs (carbimazole), iodine and beta blockers. A primary condition is when the thyroid alone is affected. In a secondary condition, the pituitary is affected and over- or under-produces TSH, which in turn affects the thyroid.

## Hypothyroidism

Hypothyroidism is low thyroid production, often with a reduced basal metabolic rate and weight gain. Most cases are primary Hashimoto's autoimmune, which destroys the thyroid tissue. As discussed earlier, some other autoimmune conditions, such as pernicious anaemia, raise auto-antibodies against the thyroid. Physical and chemical damage from trauma and radiation, as well as inappropriate sex hormone signals (sometimes seen in endometriosis) can also reduce T4 production.

## Table 11.1: Sample thyroid function test results

| TRH Hypothalamus | TSH Pituitary | T4 Thyroid | Observation |
|---|---|---|---|
| Normal | Normal | Low | Primary |
| Normal | Low | Low | Secondary |
| Low | Low | Low | Tertiary |

## Thyroid treatments

T4 medication can take between four and six weeks to affect and stabilise TSH, and this would be the optimum time after which to repeat the TFT. If too much T4 is given, this will suppress the hypothalamus, and free T4 after six weeks will be very low. The usual range for T4 is 12.0–23.0pmol/L, and for TSH it is 0.4–5.0mU/L. Therefore a TSH of under 0.01mU/L usually indicates over-replacement; and 0.01–0.4 mU/L may mean some over-replacement, especially if free T4 is >30mU/L. A TSH of 0.4–5.0mU/L usually means that the T4 replacement is sufficient, whilst a TSH of >5.0mU/L indicates probable under-replacement or patient non-compliance. This is due to the pituitary still producing high amounts of TSH to encourage the thyroid to make T4 (which it won't).

Since T4 can take up to six weeks to stabilise an adequate TSH response, patients newly commenced on thyroxine could have a repeat TFT around six to eight weeks post-intervention. Once the dose is stable, following a round of six-monthly TFT, you can then consider (if clinically appropriate) moving to an annual TFT.

Drugs such as carbimazole, normally prescribed to suppress T4 production, can be used to 'block' free T4, or they can be used as a therapy to 'block' before medicating with thyroxine to 'replace'. As with T4 supplementation for hypo-conditions, TSH levels in patients with hyper-conditions may take up to 12 weeks to respond to carbimazole. In practice, you should consider carrying out a TFT every four to six weeks, then move to every three months once stable. For other treatments, such as radioiodine, consider an interval of four to eight weeks after dose, but take clinical advice in your own healthcare setting.

# 12

## Bone profile

The bone provides skeletal structure, bone marrow production of cells, and over 99% of stored calcium (Ca). Bone is made of two structural components: the cortical (compact) and cancellous (trabecular). The cortical is the hard outer layer, making up about 80% of the bone mass. The remaining mass is mainly the trabecular, which contains blood vessels, cells and bone marrow (which makes red cells, white cells and platelets). In addition to the blood cells produced by bone marrow, bone also has two major types of cells – osteoblasts and osteoclasts. Osteoblasts mineralise bone (adding to it), whereas osteoclasts break down bone. There is another cell called an osteocyte, which is thought to modulate calcium concentration and respond to load bearing, and possibly exhibit phagocytosis.

A typical bone profile will measure calcium, phosphate, albumin, alkaline phosphatase and in some cases vitamin D and parathyroid hormone (PTH).

## Bone turnover and osteoporosis

In normal bone turnover (see Figure 12.1), the osteoclast (A) liberates Ca from the bone. This Ca is then used for metabolic processes, and over a few hours Ca levels fall. In response to this, the parathyroid gland (PTG) produces PTH and the kidney releases calcitriol (Vit $D_3$), originally derived from vitamin D in diet and skin via exposure to ultraviolet (UV) rays in the sunlight. Given the key role of the kidney-derived vitamin $D_3$ in this process (◄► urea and electrolytes or U&Es), a patient with dysfunctional renal output (as shown by a reduced estimated glomerular filtration rate (eGFR) of less than 60) may be less able to resolve a fracture and may be more predisposed to bone conditions. The PTH/VitD$_3$ complex induces increased osteoclast activity in the bone, enhances Ca uptake in the gut and increases reabsorption of Ca in the kidney. The increased calcium (as a result of the PTH/VitD$_3$ complex) is reabsorbed into the bone by the osteoblasts (B). The speed and frequency of this process is partly suppressed by the action of the hormone oestrogen (green circle).

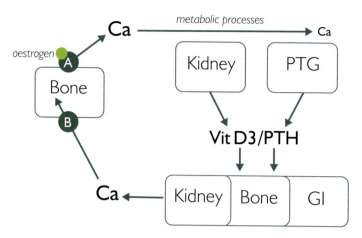

Figure 12.1: Normal bone turnover

In post-menopausal patients or those receiving long-term anti-oestrogen/progesterone treatments, this process is less regulated and more likely to result in frequent fractures, as the bone remodelling increases. This condition is called osteoporosis, and initial pre-menopausal bone mineral density (which is in turn controlled by diet, lifestyle and genetics) is an important factor in disease risk and progression. As the process is speeded up, variations in the blood components are difficult to observe. Thus, bone profile is not usually used in practice to diagnose or monitor osteoporosis. In elderly patients with chronic kidney disease, osteoporosis can be exacerbated. In addition to not being able to sustain $VitD_3$ production, these individuals have compromised reabsorption of Ca, which increases their risk of fracture and the time needed for any fractures to heal.

## Paget's disease

In Paget's disease there is a dysfunctional regulation of the osteoclast and osteoblast pathway. This leads to imperfect removal and reabsorption of Ca.

**Analogy: Imagine repairing a road. Team A (osteoclasts) remove two buckets of rubble (Ca) from the road (bone) and dispose of the Ca by using it to make muscle, nerves and teeth. But they tell Team B that they have taken out 20 buckets of rubble. The foreman (PTH) therefore insists that Team B (osteoblasts) use 20 buckets to refill the hole (even though there is only room for two buckets of rubble). Thus, the road will not return to its original flat surface. Instead, a bump will be left.**

In practice, this process leads to bone protrusions and pain. A raised Ca level is sometimes seen in patients with immobility due to joint degradation, as the sockets and joints are ill formed.

Drugs like bisphosphonates work by binding to calcium in the bone, which then suppresses osteoclast activity, thus improving and maintaining bone mineral density. Bisphosphonates are therefore often used to treat osteoporosis and Paget's.

## Osteomalacia

Patients with a vitamin D deficiency can be predisposed to osteomalacia, known as rickets in children. Vitamin D is obtained from the diet and stored in the skin. There, under the action of UV light, it is converted into vitamin $D_2$ (calcidiol), which is stored in the liver. Vitamin $D_2$ is then transported to the kidney, where it is converted, by a parathyroid hormone (PTH) induced enzyme, into vitamin $D_3$ (calcitriol 1,25 $(OH)_2D$). Inadequate production of vitamin $D_3$ often results in hypocalcaemia, leading to dysfunctional bone remodelling and eventually weak bones that 'bend' under the weight of the trunk. Causes of vitamin $D_3$ deficiency may be a lack of UV light, too little vitamin D in the diet, or the presence of chemicals in the diet that can block vitamin $D_3$ absorption in the gut (seek advice from dietetics), or renal impairment as in chronic kidney disease. Blood test results in osteomalacia are often low Ca, high PTH, as the parathyroid attempts to correct the low Ca, and low phosphate, as PTH increases excretion in the urine (◀▶ eGFR for renal status).

## Magnesium

Other tests that may be returned are magnesium (Mg), alkaline phosphatase and phosphate. Magnesium is required to produce PTH so a magnesium deficiency will restrict PTH and thus the availability of free Ca. Hypomagnesaemia is common is alcoholic patients, due to malnutrition, diarrhoea and increased excretion; the latter is also seen in diabetic keto-acidosis. Some thiazide and loop diuretics, antibiotics, proton pump inhibitors, pancreatitis and gastrointestinal (GI) disorders (such as Crohn's) may also lead to low Mg levels.

## Alkaline phosphatase

Alkaline phosphatase (Alk Phos) is an enzyme found within the bone, liver, kidney and placenta and is a helpful differential. For example, if a patient has a raised Alk Phos under the LFT, but all other LFT values are normal (as are the U&Es), this could suggest that the cause of the raised Alk Phos could be bone – especially with a raised Ca.

**Patient 4** is taking potassium-sparing diuretics or KCl supplements.

**Patient 5** has renal dysfunction and thus cannot excrete potassium effectively.

**Patient 6** is taking ACE inhibitors, ibuprofen and an antibiotic. All of these could interfere with the urinary excretion of potassium.

**Patient 7** has a mineralocorticoid deficiency, such as Addison's disease.

For all of the above patients, additional tests such as HbA1c (diabetes), pH, bicarbonate (acid base), hormone screening (adrenal, pituitary), Na, Urea (renal), LFTs (liver), full blood count (sickle cell and other blood disorders), as well as MRI scans, ECGs and patient histories, can help differentiate.

One of the treatments for acute hyperkalaemia involves shunting the potassium back into the cells. This can be done by using a dose of insulin, bicarbonate or a 2-selective catecholamine (such as salbutamol), as clinically appropriate.

Whilst Na and K are helpful in determining electrolyte and water balance, urea and cotinine are useful in order to specify a pre-, true and post-renal location, and to assess acute versus chronic conditions.

## Urea and creatinine

Creatinine is a product of muscle turnover and is a marker of chronic renal failure, demonstrating prolonged damage to the nephrons. A renal stone or a prolonged urinary tract infection (UTI) may slightly increase creatine over time.

Urea is produced from the breakdown of protein, and is cleared via the urea cycle, which controls nitrogen stores in the body. In practice, it is commonly used as a marker of acute renal dysfunction. As discussed earlier, urea can rise sharply in acute dehydration, and also as an artefact following the intake of a high protein meal. Urea levels rise in acute renal dysfunction due to renal stones, viral infection and prostate cancer.

**Patient 1** is a 70-year-old man with a history of lower back pain and infrequent urine production. He is almost anuriac. His urea, Na, and Alk Phos were all significantly raised. This could have been due to a renal stone, or UTI. Dehydration is unlikely, given the increased Alk Phos. However, a significantly increased prostate specific antigen (PSA) revealed an underlying prostatic tumour, with raised Ca and Alk Phos results from a bone profile, suggesting bone metastasis. On initial presentation to primary care, given that the patient had had a prostatectomy, prostate cancer was not thought to be likely.

**Patient 2** is a 35-year-old woman with lower back, pelvic and abdominal pain. Her U&Es were normal, so CA-125 was performed. CA-125 is highly correlated with ovarian cancer, with about 80% accuracy. It is also linked to very severe endometriosis. Following a laparoscopy, this was indeed diagnosed.

The urea:creatinine ratio can commonly be used to determine the site of renal failure and for suspected gastric bleeds. To work this out, you should first take the median (middle) value of the reference range for both urea and creatinine. In this example, the units have been standardised to $\mu$mmol/L, the range of urea is 3000–8300 and creatine is 40–130. The medians are therefore 5650 for urea and 85 for creatinine, which is a baseline value of 66:1. To help remember the distinction between creatine and creatinine, think about the test for kidney function, U&E or Ewes and Knees; this has an 'n' sound, as does creatinine (found in the kidney).

In pre-renal dysfunction, such as arterial stenosis, congestive heart failure or dehydration, urea reabsorption is increased and the U:C ratio will favour urea <100:1. A U:C of 40–100:1 (normal) is usually seen in post-renal obstructions. In true renal damage, urea reabsorption is compromised and the U:C ratio will be 1–40:1.

**Patient 3** is a child with an upper gastrointestinal (GI) bleed and an expected U:C may be 30–40:1.

The overall renal function can be monitored by testing estimated glomerular filtration rate (eGFR). The rate is 'estimated' because, unlike an actual GFR (which involves urine collection), eGFR is measured using only blood. The glomerulus is a structure within the kidney, which connects the vasculature and renal architecture and provides an initial filter for large proteins and cells. **Analogy: The glomerulus is a bit like a sieve filled with cotton wool, under a running tap.**

A normal eGFR is around 100ml/min. But age, even without specific disease pathology, affects the glomerulus. From the age of about 35, the eGFR value falls by about 10% per decade. It may therefore be 'normal' for an 80-year-old patient to have an 'abnormal' eGFR of 60. However, an eGFR of 60 in a 19-year-old would be more worrying. Since eGFR is based on creatinine clearance (and thus muscle turnover), patients with an African or Caribbean heritage, or with a large muscle mass, should consider having their eGFR adjusted by multiplying by 1.2.

## Glomerular filtration rate

The eGFR forms the basis for chronic kidney disease (CKD) staging and sets the scene for a differential or adjunct diagnosis where renal function can affect the pathology, such as COPD, acid base, anaemia, vitamin D deficiency, diabetes and so on. In clinical practice, an eGFR

>60mL/min is usually adequate. Some laboratories will therefore not return a numerical value if greater than this and simply report eGFR >60. Some may give numerical values, and more commonly a narrative about CKD status. However, there is some debate about the clinical relevance of some mild staging, particularly in the elderly, for the reasons discussed above.

## Table 13.1: CKD stages and eGFR values

| eGFR value | CKD stage |
|---|---|
| >90 | 1: Normal |
| >60 | 2: Mild |
| >30 | 3: Moderate; less reversible |
| >15 | 4: Severe |
| <15 | 5: Established; consider dialysis or transplantation |

## Urate and gout

Urate or uric acid is often raised in patients with gout. Urate is a breakdown product of cellular metabolism, and – more specifically – DNA breakdown. Urate is held in the blood as soluble crystal. However, if the levels of urate rise or a renal impairment affects blood volume and flow (or both), it will quickly precipitate out of solution and form a solid crystal, usually at the interphalangeal joints of the toes. **Analogy: Imagine floating sticks down a shallow river that is flowing over rocks. The more sticks (urate) you throw in, the more likely they are to get stuck. Also, if the level of the river (blood volume or flow) falls, the sticks will get stuck amongst the rocks.**

Urate levels can be raised through poor diet, chemicals called purines and eating food high in DNA such as liver and pâté. High urate may also be seen in leukaemia patients due to the high DNA turnover in the breakdown of large numbers of white blood cells. (◀▶ gout to FBC: WBC.) However, in view of the inflammation, a rise in white blood cell count (WBC) and inflammatory markers may be expected.

Renal impairment, with an eGFR less than 60mL/min may predispose a patient to gout. Raised Ca may be an indication of pseudo-gout, especially if the gout is non-responsive to allopurinal (which blocks urate production). A comparison of the crystal structure will provide a helpful differential.

# 14

# Liver function tests

The liver has three key functions: storage (◀▶ deficiencies in iron, $B_{12}$ and glucose); metabolic production (◀▶ production of cholesterol, CRP, fibrinogen (PT, INR, aPTT) and albumin); and detoxification of endogenous and exogenous toxins. Liver function tests (LFTs) will usually report enzymes, albumin and bilirubin levels. If the test name ends in 'ase' or has the units (IU/L) then it is an enzyme. An enzyme takes a substrate (usually not soluble and toxic) and converts it into a product (usually more soluble and less toxic).

Almost all enzymes are intracellular. The presence of high concentrations of enzymes in the blood means that cells have been destroyed, allowing the enzymes to 'leak out'. Possible causes of cellular destruction could be trauma, alcoholic cirrhosis, viral damage from hepatitis, or cellular necrosis (cell death) resulting from drug toxicity. The particular enzymes raised will usually indicate which type of damage has occurred.

A standard LFT may contain:

- Bilirubin: Plumbing of the liver – pre-, actual, post- and red blood cell turnover
- Alanine aminotransferase (ALT): Viral hepatitis and drug toxicity – refer to British National Formulary (see Further Reading, page 76) and the pharmacy department in your local healthcare setting
- Aspartate aminotransferase (AST): Alcoholic hepatitis, acute liver failure
- Alkaline phosphatase (ALP or Alk Phos): The biliary tree, gall stones, pancreas
- Gamma-glutamyltransferase (GGT): Alcohol, analgesics and opiates
- Amylase: Pancreatitis
- Albumin: Decreased on liver failure
- International normalised ratio (INR): Now being used as a surrogate liver marker. In liver failure, fibrinogen production is compromised, and clotting time (INR) is therefore significantly extended.

As the liver is a dynamic and interconnected organ, the blood results from the LFT may be difficult to interpret when presented as a list on a results screen or printout. Instead, it may be helpful to imagine them superimposed onto a general anatomy and physiology diagram, and interconnected to other organs.

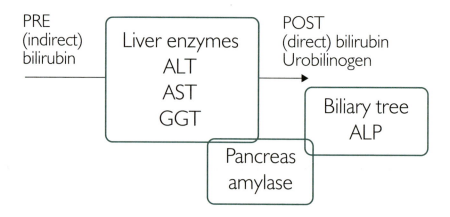

Figure 14.1: Liver enzymes

# Bilirubin

Bilirubin is a breakdown product of red blood cells. Elevated bilirubin is called jaundice, and bilirubin is a marker of 'plumbing' in the liver. Pre-hepatic bilirubin is called indirect or unconjugated. In the liver an enzyme called UGT1A1 (which is dysfunctional in Gilbert's syndrome) converts indirect bilirubin into direct, or conjugated bilirubin. The conjugated bilirubin is then partly used to produce urobilinogen and partly excreted in the faeces. The LFT result of 'Total bilirubin' is direct + indirect, both of which can also be measured to further investigate liver dysfunction. As indirect bilirubin rises, this is usually a pre- or actual hepatic condition; a rise in the direct form usually indicates a post-hepatic blockage.

Jaundice can occur when high levels of bilirubin are produced in polycythaemia (◄► full blood count and red blood cell count). High levels of bilirubin from the red cells overload the liver and may predispose the patient to jaundice. Jaundice can also be seen in actual liver damage, with high liver enzyme concentrations of aspartate aminotransferase (AST), alanine aminotransferase (ALT) and gamma-glutamyltransferase (GGT). Often bilirubin rises before the liver enzymes do. This may occur in patients undergoing chemotherapy, or those with hepatitis (both viral and alcoholic), or being treated with antibiotics or with some genetic conditions. In a post-hepatic blockage (with high Alk phos/amylase and raised liver enzymes) bilirubin will increase and this can be linked to the absence of urobilinogen.

# Aminotransferases

Alanine aminotransferase (ALT) is a liver enzyme that closely reflects chronic and acute liver damage. It is often raised in viral hepatitis, drug toxicity or overdose.

Aspartate aminotransferase (AST) is a liver enzyme that indicates acute liver damage. It is often raised in alcoholic patients, due to severe liver damage. It can be used in conjunction with ALT to assess the extent of liver dysfunction.

In a raised ALT, you should ask the following:

* Is the value more than 1.5 x above the upper range?
* Is the patient symptomatic?
* Are bilirubin, INR and albumin also abnormal?

If the answer to any of these questions is 'yes', further investigations should be considered. If the answer is 'no', then consider repeating the test.

In the following examples, the upper reference range for AST is 38IU/L and for ALT 41IU/L. The figures used demonstrate which enzyme is raised, and should not be used as a diagnostic cut-off in practice.

**Patient 1** has AST 100IU/L and ALT 22IU/L, and all other LFTs are normal. AST is also found in cardiac tissue so investigation of chest pain may reveal a cardiac event.

**Patient 2** has ALT 100IU/L and AST 48IU/L, which could indicate viral hepatitis, toxicity to methotrexate, or over-use of analgesics.

**Patient 3** is an alcoholic patient with severe liver damage. AST is 200IU/L and ALT is 100IU/L. If the AST was to increase to 500IU/L the prognosis would become increasingly poor.

**Patient 4** has obstetric cholestasis, presenting with pruritus (itch) and raised ALT. Bile salts are ordered. Bile salts are made by the liver and stored in the gall bladder; they are then secreted into the duodenum to dissolve fats (enterohepatic circulation). In hepatobiliary conditions, the enterohepatic circulation is dysfunctional and bile salts can be secreted into the systemic circulation. Given the lipid-dissolving, surfactant properties of bile salts, their presence in a pregnant patient's systemic circulation could lead to foetal distress or damage.

# Gamma-glutamyltransferase (GGT)

The enzyme gamma-glutamyltransferase (GGT) is often used as a marker for alcohol intake. GGT can be elevated for up to five days following alcohol intake. However, ◀▶ full blood count (FBC) and the mean cell volume (MCV) because a raised GGT could be due to transient alcohol intake. A high GGT and a folate-deficient macrocytic anaemia, caused by alcohol intake, are more indicative of alcohol abuse. As this will take at least 6–12 weeks to develop, consider the red blood cell lifespan.

## Alkaline phosphatase

The enzyme alkaline phosphatase (Alk phos or ALP) is also present in other organs (bones, kidney and placenta) so ◀▶ these tests, symptoms and history. Liver-specific Alk phos is an enzyme mainly found in the cells that line the bile ducts and biliary tree. Therefore ALP is usually elevated with bile duct blockage – caused by gall stones, pancreatitis, post-hepatic tumour or cholestasis.

If ALP is raised and GGT is not, then consider a non-hepatic condition. If GGT is raised, and/or ALP is twice the upper range, and/or both ALP and GGT have been raised for more than three months, and/or the patient has symptoms, consider a liver ultrasound.

## Amylase

The enzyme amylase is found in the pancreas and saliva. It is therefore often elevated in pancreatitis.

**Patient 5** had a rise in amylase (pancreas), bilirubin (post-hepatic blockage) and Alk phos (biliary tree), followed by GGT, ALT and then AST (secondary liver damage), which represented the progression of a pancreatic tumour.

## Albumin

Albumin is a protein made by the liver and has three main roles: as a chaperone (transporter) for molecules like calcium (◀▶ bone profile); to provide pressure and osmotic stability in the blood, and is thus linked to oedema and renal function (◀▶ U&Es); and as a precursor for antibody production (globulins). Albumin can also be decreased in malnutrition, but other LFTs are likely to be normal. Since albumin is made by the liver, any dysfunction will probably reduce albumin concentrations (hypoalbuminaemia). However, you should check the U&Es as some renal dysfunction will not retain albumin, and proteins and cells are likely to be present in the urine.

## Alcohol and drug abuse, and viral infection

**Patient 6** has raised aminotransferases (>300IU/L), due to a viral infection and paracetamol overdose, in addition to an alcoholic liver disease.

As the viral infection becomes acute, this value may rise higher still. An AST >400IU/L and a peak ALT of 1000IU/L is associated with severe liver damage due to paracetamol overdose. For the hepatitis viral infection in practice, this can also be seen in the diagnosis of viral hepatitis. Hepatitis B surface antigen (HepBsAg) may indicate a current infection. Alternatively, a new, rapid technique is to measure the DNA or RNA of the HepB virus directly in the cell.

Patients who use cocaine, marijuana or heroin alone will usually have out-of-range LFTs, including AST and GGT. If injecting, a raised ALT may often indicate a viral hepatitis. If the patient is alcoholic (raised MCV and raised GGT), additional drug use will also affect these measures.

**Analogy: Imagine that the liver function test is a pirate's treasure map.**

**Bilirubin, the grumpy pirate from the red cell, is brought to the island (liver) and paired up with another grumpy bilirubin pirate by the island's dating agency (the enzyme UGT1A1). The two are now happy as a pair and leave the island via the biliary tree. Hence, we can map bilirubin to pre, actual and post hepatic blockage by counting up how many single (indirect bilirubin) or paired pirates (direct bilirubin) we have.**

**The liver island is made up of special cages (hepatocyte liver cells) which hold animals (enzymes) called AST, GGT and ALT. If the cages (cells) are damaged then the animals will escape the island and be found in large numbers in the sea (blood), suggesting a problem with the island.**

**The island's factories make albumin and fibrinogen; if the island is damaged then the amounts of these will fall.**

**The liver island has neighbouring smaller islands (gall bladder and pancreas) connected by diamond (ALP) encrusted bridges (the biliary tree). The gall bladder has a rich diamond reserve (ALP) and only the pancreas island has coconuts (amylase).**

**Thus, if the pancreas island was damaged, the sea would probably contain:**
- **Coconuts (ALP), from the damaged pancreas island**
- **Diamonds (ALP), with the pancreas island damaged, the bridges to this island are now overwhelmed with the products made by the liver island trying to get out, and thus these bridges are damaged.**

- **Paired Grumpy Pirates, the liver island has paired the pirates but with the bridges out broken they will increase in number.**
- **Freed animals (ALT and GGT and AST), given that the exit route is blocked over time the liver island will be damaged and so the cages holding the animals will break open.**

# Afterword

In this book I have tried to help you:

- Appreciate the importance of blood tests in diagnosis and patient management
- Increase your current knowledge by defining what each test is, and explaining what it shows from a physiological and biochemical viewpoint
- Understand the many abbreviations used in blood tests
- Determine the clinical significance of values outside the reference range, or indeed an ill person with normal results
- Develop linking of tests and using tests for exclusion
- Work through the strategy example in Chapter 2, adapting it to your own clinical setting
- Explore how tests form a natural hierarchy, with full blood count (FBC), urea and electrolytes (U&Es) and liver function tests (LFTs) being common first-line tests, which may then justify more specific (and often more expensive) tests.

The book also introduces various analogies and metaphors to aid memory and understanding, in addition to the usual scientific or clinical definitions. The analogies have been tested in a variety of settings and I hope they have helped you understand the concepts and given you some ideas as to how you can explain these issues to patients who ask about blood tests. Clearly, many of the analogies are significantly simplified for the sake of clarity. You could also try to create metaphors of your own, and I would be very interested to hear about them on **Twitter: @grahambasten**

Good luck!

# Further reading and references

## Books and articles

Ahmed, N. (2010). *Clinical Biochemistry*. Oxford: Oxford University Press.

Bratt-Wyton, R. (1998). Interpretation of routine blood tests. *Nursing Standard*. **13**:12, 42–48.

Higgins, C. (2007). *Understanding Laboratory Investigations: For Nurses and Health Professionals*. Oxford: Wiley-Blackwell.

Knight, R. (2012). *Transfusion and Transplantation Science*. Oxford: Oxford University Press.

Luxton, R. (2008). *Clinical Biochemistry*. Banbury, Oxfordshire: Scion.

Pallister, C. & Watson, M. (2010). *Haematology*. Banbury, Oxfordshire: Scion.

Skinner, S. (1995). *Understanding Clinical Investigations: A Quick Reference Manual*. Oxford: Baillière Tindall.

## Internet resources

**Arthritis Research UK**
http://www.arthritisresearchuk.org/

**BD Vacutainer Tube Guide**
http://www.bd.com/vacutainer/

**BookBoon**
http://bookboon.com/en/textbooks/biology-biochemistry/introduction-to-clinical-biochemistry
Search 'Basten'

**British Committee for Standards in Haematology**
http://www.bcshguidelines.com/

**British National Formulary**
http://www.bnf.org/

**British Thyroid Foundation**
http://www.btf-thyroid.org/

Diabetes UK
http://www.diabetes.org.uk/

Health and Care Professions Council (HCPC)
http://www.hpc-uk.org/

Institute of Biomedical Science (IBMS)
http://www.ibms.org/

Lab Tests Online (apps for tablet devices and smart phones, based on USA data)
http://www.labtestsonline.org.uk/

Leeds Pathology
http://www.pathology.leedsth.nhs.uk/Pathology/

NHS Choices
http://www.nhs.uk/Pages/HomePage.aspx

NICE Guidelines
http://www.nice.org.uk/guidance/index.jsp?action=byType&type=2&status=3

NICE Pathways
http://pathways.nice.org.uk/

Nursing and Midwifery Council (NMC)
http://www.nmc-uk.org/

Nursing Times
http://www.nursingtimes.net/

Royal College of Nursing (RCN)
http://www.rcn.org.uk/

# Index